Editors
G. TORSELLO - K. P

Contributors

M. Austermann	M. Lachat
B. Berekoven	F. Marques de Azevedo
T. Bisdas	G. Panuccio

ENDOVASCULAR TREATMENT OF COMPLEX ABDOMINAL AND THORACOABDOMINAL ANEURYSMS

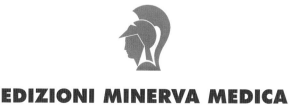

EDIZIONI MINERVA MEDICA

This book is dedicated to Roy K. Greenberg,
who continues to inspire us to push the limits
of endovascular treatment of aortic pathologies.

ISBN: 978-88-7711-755-7

FOREWORD

Until a few years ago, open surgery was the only form of treatment for patients with aortic pathologies. However, less invasive methods such as endografting with chimney, branched and fenestrated stent grafts have been increasing in importance in recent years. The demographic changes and the increasing number of high-risk patients have led to a shift toward endovascular techniques. This book focuses on illustrating the alternative techniques to open surgery for treatment of complex aortic diseases in high-risk patients.

Some of the techniques, *e.g.* the use of fenestrated grafts, were introduced more than ten years ago. Accordingly, long-term results of this technique are available; benefits as well as limitations of this technique are well-known.

Other procedures such as the chimney technique are relatively new and not yet standardized. Mid- and long-term follow up results are still not available. Initially used as a bail-out procedure, the technique is now discussed as an alternative treatment of patients with extremely short or no aneurysm neck.

As thoracoabdominal aortic aneurysms still represent one of the most demanding pathologies with high morbidity and mortality, even in specialized cardiovascular centers, the description of the complete endovascular approach with branched endografts and the hybrid techniques will have a central role in this book.

All possible approaches at the present day are described in a step-by-step manner, including complications and trouble shooting procedures. I would like to point out that the informations presented in this book are based on our many years of clinical experience, and may not entirely align with recommendations of the device manufacturers. Refer to the manufacturer's instructions for use for specific information on a device.

I thank the authors for their contribution and Priya Bharadwaj, Ph. D., Jennifer McCann-Brown, Ph.D., and Jarin Kratzberg, Ph.D., for technical review.

I hope the book is helpful in your practice to choose a tailored strategy in sense of a case-to-case oriented treatment of complex aortic diseases.

GIOVANNI TORSELLO

List of Contributors

EDITORS

GIOVANNI TORSELLO, MD
Department of Vascular Surgery, Münster University Hospital and St. Franziskus Hospital Münster, Münster, Germany

KONSTANTINOS P. DONAS, MD
Department of Vascular Surgery, Münster University Hospital and St. Franziskus Hospital Münster, Münster, Germany

CONTRIBUTORS

MARTIN AUSTERMANN, MD
Department of Vascular Surgery, St. Franziskus Hospital Münster, Münster, Germany

MARIO LACHAT, MD
Clinic of Cardiovascular Surgery, Zurich University Hospital, Zurich, Switzerland

THEODOSIOS BISDAS, MD
Department of Vascular Surgery, Münster University Hospital, Münster, Germany

GIUSEPPE PANUCCIO, MD
Department of Vascular Surgery, Münster University Hospital, Münster, Germany

BÄRBEL BEREKOVEN
Department of Vascular Surgery, St. Franziskus Hospital Münster, Münster, Germany

FRANCISCO MARQUES DE AZEVEDO
Department of Vascular Surgery, St. Franziskus Hospital Münster, Münster, Germany

Contents

Abbreviations

BECS: balloon expandable covered stent

CIA: common iliac artery

CSF: cerebro spinal fluid

CT: celiac trunk

EIA: external iliac artery

F: French

IBD: iliac branch device

IIA: internal iliac artery

LRA: left renal artery

LSA: left subclavian artery

RRA: right renal artery

SMA: superior mesenteric artery

SECS: self expandable covered stent

CHAPTER 1

The chimney endovascular technique

K.P. Donas, G. Torsello, M. Austermann

Endovascular aortic aneurysm repair of challenging anatomies is technically demanding and potentially hazardous. The main concern is inadequate endograft sealing, especially in short necks. The chimney endovascular technique has been primarily suggested as a rescue procedure for over-stented aortic side branches during endovascular treatment; however, it has also been used to increase the sealing zone in cases of an insufficient neck for endovascular approach.

There is no consensus or recommendation in the current literature about the suitable type of chimney grafts. Generally, balloon expandable covered stents (BECS), such as the Advanta/i-Cast, are characterized by high radial force and good fluoroscopic visibility, which allows for precise placement of the bridging devices in the target vessels. The Advanta stent-graft shows advanced conformability and adaptability of the device in the target vessel. Additional placement of a self-expanding bare stent increases the flexibility of the BECS, but placing the additional component in the small diameter target vessels may provoke significant reduction of the patent lumen and subsequent occlusion. In this context, the new generation of the Advanta/i-Cast (Atrium) covered stents, characterized by an open cell design (Figure 1.1), aims to improve the flexibility of the Advanta/i-Cast stent-grafts without reducing the radial force.

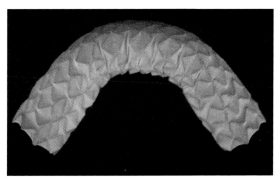

Figure 1.1 The new generation of the Advanta/iCast balloon-expandable covered stent with open-cell design.

Importantly, the chimney technique is feasible with the majority of available abdominal endografts. This fact allows urgent endovascular treatment of symptomatic or ruptured aneurysms with abdominal endoprostheses available in stock at any vascular center. Flexible devices with low profiles, such as the Endurant stent graft (Medtronic), perform very well in combination with BECS also in case with severe calcification and tortuosity in the iliacs, which may be very hazardous for fenestrated endografting.

Coscas *et al.* reported extensively on the issue of the "gutters", also known as perigraft channels, located between the aorta, the chimneys and the abdominal endograft. The "gutters" might be the origin of type Ia endoleaks. However, the current published literature showed that occurrence of type Ia endoleak is rare. They can also be treated by cuff implantation or glue embolization (Onyx; ev3).

Indications and limitations

Anatomical preconditions for the use of chimney technique are the presence of at least a 15 mm neck distance between the target vessel which needs chimney graft implantation and the first aortic side branch above the covered stent. Other important prerequisites are patent subclavian artery and absence of extensive thrombus in the aortic arch and suprarenal segment. In cases where more than two branches of the pararenal aortic pathology are involved, fenestrated endografts should also be considered.

Procedure

- Cut down or puncture of the brachial artery and device/graft/stent introduction over a 0.035 Terumo wire (Terumo) and a 5 F catheter (MPA or Headhunter). In case of multiple chimneys, contralateral access is additionally required. Alternatively, cut down of the subclavian artery can be performed. Suturing of a large external conduit facilitates access, avoiding trauma to the subclavian artery.
- Catheterization of the target vessel. Withdrawal of the guide wire and application of contrast medium to exclude dissection and to identify side branches of the target vessel (Figure 1.2 A).

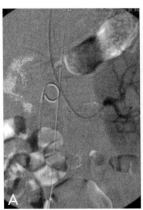 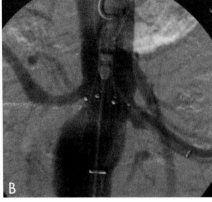

Figure 1.2 A) Digital subtraction angiography after catheterization of the target vessel to ensure the intraluminal positioning of the system. B) The 7 F-sheath is advanced and positioned in the target vessel (left renal artery). The main body of the abdominal stent graft has been partially deployed covering the origin of the left renal artery.

- Introduction of the Rosen wire (Cook), which has a tight less traumatic J tip over a 6 F or 7 F shuttle sheath (Cook) into the target vessel. The sheath is placed into the target vessel. After this, the main body of the abdominal endograft can be partially deployed at the origin of the left renal artery (Figure 1.2 B).
- Figure 1.3 A shows a juxtarenal aortic aneurysm with the SMA and left renal artery origins at the same level. The right renal artery has a chronic occlusion. In planning the implantation of two chimney grafts in two different target vessels, as in this case, bilateral puncture or cut down of the brachial artery is necessary. In a similar manner to that previously described for one chimney graft, two 7 F sheaths are placed in the SMA and left renal artery over the Rosen wire. This allows for advancement and partial deployment of the abdominal stent-graft with covering of the origin of the target vessels (Figure 1.3 B). The goal is to create a minimum neck length of 10 mm.
- Abdominal endograft placement follows the insertion of the chimney graft (Advanta V12, Atrium) in the target vessel. After retraction of the sheath, the chimney graft can be deployed (Figure 1.4). We recommend at least a 2 cm landing zone for the chimney graft into the target vessel. The end of the chimney graft has to be between the covered part of the abdominal endograft and the anchor pins or hooks.

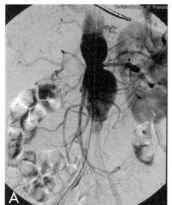
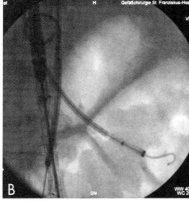

Figure 1.3 A) Juxtarenal aortic aneurysm with origin of the superior mesenteric artery and left renal artery at the same level. The right renal artery is chronic occluded. B) Successful placement of the 7-sheaths over Rosen wires in the SMA and left renal artery. The abdominal stent-graft is partially deployed at the origin of the target vessels.

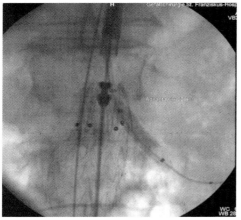

Figure 1.4 The placement and full expansion of the abdominal endograft follows the deployment of the chimney graft in the target vessel (left renal artery).

TIP: in cases of an unstable positioning of the sheath, we suggest to have the covered stent already in the estimated location within the target vessel at the end of the sheath. Disadvantage of this maneuver may be that the length of the covered stent has to be previously determined.

TIP: in cases of chimney graft implantation, an oblique angiography in the renal arteries is helpful to document the origin of the SMA. This can prevent an inadvertent over-stenting of the SMA.

- Placement of bare stents in order to "reline" the chimney graft is optional.
- Kissing PTA of chimney graft and abdominal endograft: the chimney graft has to be inflated first, then the abdominal endograft; otherwise, fracture or collapse of the chimney graft is possible, especially when balloon expandable covered stents are used. Figure 1.5 illustrates the kissing PTA maneuver in one case with multiple chimneys (*i.e.* SMA and left renal artery) between the aortic endograft and the chimney grafts. Figure 1.6 demonstrates the final result of a single chimney graft deployed in the left renal artery with synchronous placement of the abdominal endograft at the origin of the target vessel. In this case, a bare stent (SMART, Cordis) for relining of the chimney graft was also implanted within the covered stent providing flexibility.

TIP: additional placement of bare stents within the chimney grafts may lead to significant narrow of the patent lumen of small target vessels with consecutive occlusion.

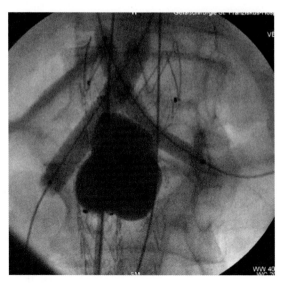

Figure 1.5 Kissing PTA maneuver in case of multiple chimney grafts (i.e. superior mesenteric artery, left renal artery; the right renal artery was chronic occluded) between the chimney grafts and the aortic endograft.

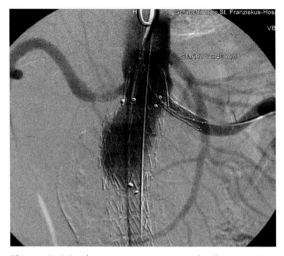

Figure 1.6 Final intraoperative angiography showing patent chimney graft and successful treatment of the aneurysm with absence of endoleak.

Persistent type I endoleak

The chimney endovascular technique can be also used in cases of a rapidly growing abdominal aortic aneurysm caused by dislocation of a previously implanted abdominal endograft.

The case presented in Figure 1.7 A demonstrates a 10 cm abdominal aortic aneurysm after previous implantation of a Talent endoprosthesis in a patient with severe iliac and neck angulation. The Talent endograft migrated, resulting in type IA (proximal) and IB (distal) endoleaks. The patient was treated by implantation of Endurant cuffs and a chimney stent-graft for the right renal artery (extending the proximal fixation of the endograft) and an Endurant limb (for distal extension of the right Talent limb) (Figure 1.7 B).

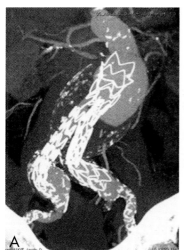
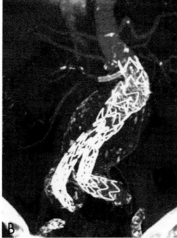

Figure 1.7 A) Proximal (Ia) and distal (Ib) endoleak caused by migration of a previous implanted Talent stent-graft. B) Postoperative CT angiography which demonstrates successful treatment of the type Ia and Ib endoleak. The used devices were Endurant tubes and chimney stent-graft (Advanta V12) for the right renal artery in order to extent the proximal fixation of the endograft and Endurant limb for distal extension of the right Talent limb.

References

1. Coscas R, Kobeiter H, Desgranges P, *et al.* Technical aspects, current indications, and results of chimney grafts for juxtarenal aortic aneurysms. J Vasc Surg 2011;53:1520-7.
2. Donas KP, Pecoraro F, Torsello G, *et al.* Use of covered chimney stents for pararenal aortic pathologies is safe and feasible with excellent patency and low incidence of endoleaks J Vasc Surg 2012;55:659-65.
3. Donas KP, Torsello G, Austermann M, *et al.* Use of abdominal chimney grafts is safe and feasible. Short-term results. J Endovasc Ther 2010;17:589-93.
4. Ohrlander T, Sonesson B, Ivancev K, *et al.* The chimney graft: a technique for preserving or rescuing aortic branch vessels in stent-graft sealing zones. J Endovasc Ther 2008;15:427-32.
5. Bruen KJ, Feezor RJ, Daniels MJ, *et al.* Endovascular chimney technique versus open repair of juxtarenal and suprarenal aneurysms. J Vasc Surg 2011;53:895-905.
6. Donas KP, Eisenack M, Torsello G, *et al.* The role of open and endovascular treatment with fenestrated and chimney endografts of patients with juxtarenal aortic aneurysms. J Vasc Surg 2012 [Epub ahead of print].

CHAPTER 2

The "Sandwich" technique

K.P. Donas, M. Austermann

The surgical treatment of thoracoabdominal aortic aneurysms (TAAAs) is very challenging. The "Sandwich" technique is an alternative endovascular treatment strategy which consists of deployment of one or more parallel covered stents between two endografts. The current literature provides scant information about this approach. The main indication for this technique is resolving the problem of the short length of the chimneys in cases of TAAAs with extensive involvement of the aorta. The technique may be valid in the urgent setting when a custom-made endograft cannot be used and the patient is at high-risk for open surgery (Figure 2.1). In elective cases, the technique can be considered in patients with significant tortuosity of the iliac vessels, which may lead to a hazardous branched endografting.

Limitations

For the construction of chimneys, the standard access through the subclavian artery and the aortic arch has to be feasible. Absence of floating thrombus in the aortic arch is important to avoid postoperative stroke. For the periscopes, both iliac arteries have to be patent. The main concern of this technique is the impairment of aortic flow

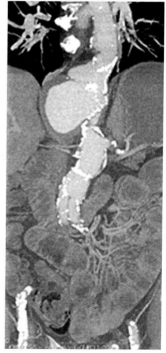

Figure 2.1 Ruptured thoracoabdominal aneurysm after previous infrarenal aortic reconstruction.

in narrow aortic lumen caused by the chimneys and periscopes. The risk is increased in patients with calcified or small aortas (*i.e.*, diameters of <16 mm), especially for periscope grafts that are perfused in a retrograde manner. Another issue is the need of high imaging tools because multiple chimneys and periscopes burden the view, making additional placement of bare stents necessary.

Procedure

- Advance and deployment of the thoracic stent-graft.
- Insertion of the covered parallel grafts has to be performed transbrachially or transaxillary in case of chimneys (Figure 2.2), as described by the chimney technique, or via transfemoral access in case of periscopes. In case of periscopes, branch cannulation can be achieved using a 45 cm sheath, a 5 F visceral reverse curve catheter over a Rosen wire (Cook).
- Use of 10 to 15 cm-long parallel grafts as chimneys or periscopes for the renovisceral arteries is necessary to obtain a long overlap zone of >5 cm with the aortic stent-graft (Figure 2.3). Usually, Viabahn (W.L. Gore) or Fluency stent-grafts (C.R. Bard) measuring 5 to 13 mm in diameter and 5 to 10 cm in length are positioned in the target arteries and deployed with the distal end inserted about 2 cm into the target vessel.
- Deployment of the aortic bridging stent-graft with long overlap zone (>5 cm) with the already placed thoracic endograft.
- A kissing balloon technique (Figure 2.4) completes the procedure by achieving full expansion of all the stent-grafts (aortic, periscopes, chimneys). In this way the chimney or periscopes grafts are "sandwiched" between the bridged aortic stent-grafts.
- A completion angiography should be per-

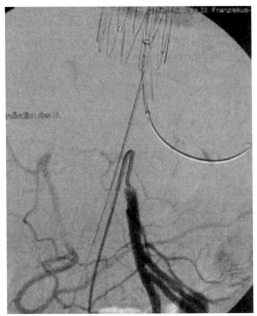

Figure 2.2 After deployment of the proximal thoracic tube graft cannulation of the superior mesenteric artery via a SOS catheter from transfemoral and of the celiac trunk via the transaxillary access using Headhunter catheter. A Rosen wire is advanced into the target vessels.

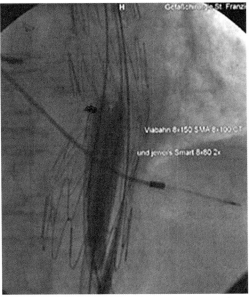

Figure 2.3 Implantation of two Viabahn stent-grafts in the visceral vessels with additional placement of two bare self-expanding stents (S.M.A.R.T; 8x80 mm) and subsequent deployment of the distal thoracic graft.

formed to exclude type I endoleak caused by persistent gutters and confirm patency of the stented visceral vessels (Figure 2.5 A,C).

In this context, it is also possible to identify postoperatively low flow type Ia endoleaks, which are due to perioperative coagulopathy in unstable patients. Postoperative pain relief is a positive clinical sign to decide for waiting and do not treat the endoleak too early. Once coagulation is normalized, the leak will disappear.

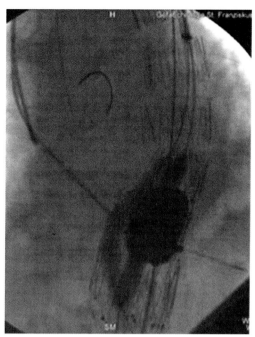

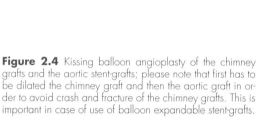

Figure 2.4 Kissing balloon angioplasty of the chimney grafts and the aortic stent-grafts; please note that first has to be dilated the chimney graft and then the aortic graft in order to avoid crash and fracture of the chimney grafts. This is important in case of use of balloon expandable stent-grafts.

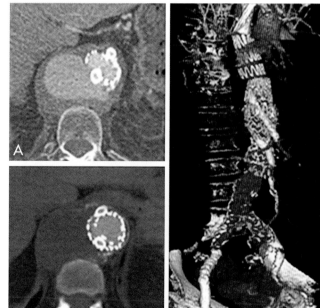

Figure 2.5 A) Angio-CT scan at discharge with evidence of type Ia endoleak caused probably by patent "gutters". B) 6-month follow-up CT scan with absence of persistent type Ia endoleak. C) CT angiography presenting the final result of the "Sandwich" technique with successful treatment of the ruptured aneurysm.

References

1. Kolvenbach RR, Yoshida R, Pinter L, *et al.* Urgent endovascular treatment of thoraco-abdominal aneurysms using a sandwich technique and chimney grafts - a technical description. Eur J Vasc Endovasc Surg 2011;41(1):54-60.

CHAPTER 3

Hybrid open endovascular procedure

K.P. Donas, M. Lachat, T. Bisdas

Treatment of pararenal (PAAAs) or thoracoabdominal (TAAAs) aortic aneurysms is challenging due to involvement of renovisceral vessels. Despite the development of many surgical strategies, the operative mortality across the United States is greater than commonly reported in the literature based on the International Classification of Diseases, Ninth Revision, Clinical Modification (ICD-9-CM) and mandates a re-examination of the treatment strategies. In contrast to the total endovascular approach, hybrid open-endovascular procedures are readily available and reproducible, avoiding aortic cross clamping and two cavities thoracoabdominal approach. However, any conclusion about the effectiveness and safety of the treatment based on the published cases remains premature; the combined approach is time consuming with a significant number of technically demanding anastomoses to the renovisceral vessels tending to bypass-related complications and failures.

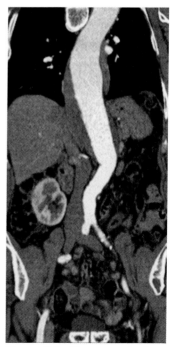

Figure 3.1 CT angiography showing a large type III thoracoabdominal aortic aneurysm of a high-risk patient with severe cardiac insufficiency.

Procedure

– Figure 3.1 shows the CT angiography of a type III TAAA. Mesenteric and renal debranching is performed from the iliac axis or distal aorta before placing an endoluminal

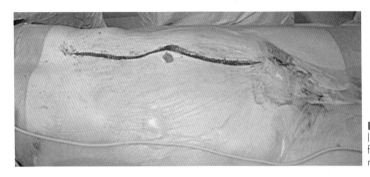

Figure 3.2 The abdominal midline incision is the standard access for hybrid repair of thoracoabdominal and pararenal aortic aneurysms.

graft designed to cover the involved aortic segment. The abdominal midline incision is the standard access for hybrid repair of TAAAs and PAAAs (Figure 3.2). Figure 3.3 shows a bifurcated Dacron bypass (14x7x7 mm), which is anastomosed with an 8 mm Dacron graft for the SMA. The two branches of the bifurcated graft are going to be used for the anastomoses to the renal arteries.

– The target vessels are exposed until a suitable bypass graft site is obtained. After heparin administration, proximal anastomosis of the prosthetic bypass (PTFE or Dacron grafts) can be performed either with the distal abdominal aorta or with the iliac arteries end-to-side. Figure 3.4 A shows the anastomoses with both renal arteries.

– Prosthetic bypass graft conduits are routed through the retroperitoneal space in case of a primary retroperitoneal approach due to hostile abdomen from the iliac arteries or transabdominally to their respective vessels. Routinely, two separate grafts for mesenteric and celiac bypass are preferred, which allows better graft orientation and anastomosed end-to-side to the target vessels. Figure 3.4 B shows the anastomosis in the hepatic artery retropancreatically. Figure 3.4 C demonstrates the final result of the renovisceral debranching, including the two renal arteries and SMA.

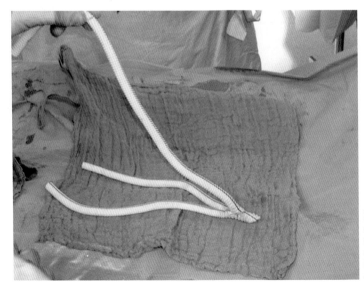

Figure 3.3 The modified bifurcated Dacron bypass graft (14x7x7 mm) for the renal arteries with the additional 8 mm Dacron bypass branch for the superior mesenteric artery or celiac trunc.

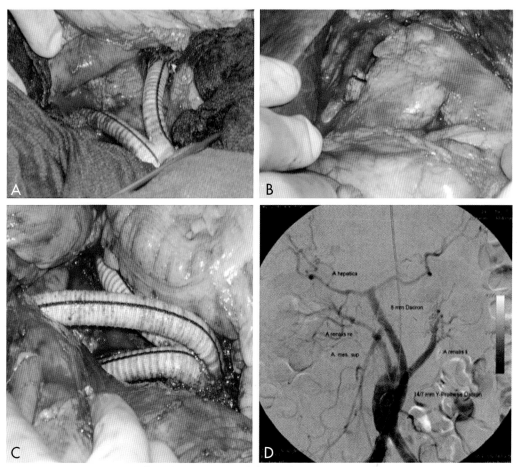

Figure 3.4 A) The already performed anastomoses with the renal arteries (intraoperative view). B) Anastomosis to the hepatic artery through retropancreatical access. C) Intraoperative status of the proximal "central" anastomosis of the modified bifurcated bypass graft to the distal abdominal aorta. D) Digital subtraction angiography of the debranching with retrograde revascularization of the renovisceral target vessels.

- The implantation of the graft to the SMA in a "lazy C" fashion can avoid potential kinking when the small bowel is returned to the abdomen. The planed limb to the celiac axis can be tunnelled in front of the renal vein through the tissue behind the pancreas, and the anastomosis can be performed to the inferior aspect of the confluence between the hepatic and left gastric arteries.
- After renovisceral debranching, the next step is the exclusion of the aneurysm by stent-graft placement. The intraoperative angiography confirms patent target vessels after debranching (Figure 3.4 D). Finally, the thoraco-abdominal stent-grafts are deployed after identification of the main feeding bypass in an oblique projection of the aortic segment (Figure 3.5 A,B). The CT angiography demonstrates an excellent result with successful debranching of the renovisceral vessels and exclusion of the aneurysm by stent-grafts placement (Figure 3.6 A,B).

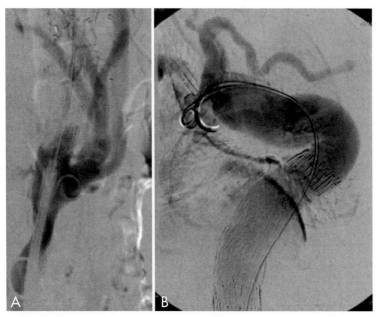

Figure 3.5 A) The distal aortic stent-graft has to be placed carefully in order to avoid covering of the main proximal anastomosis of the modified bypass. B) The placement of the aortic stent-grafts is performed in a trombone technique. The proximal aortic stent-graft was deployed successfully.

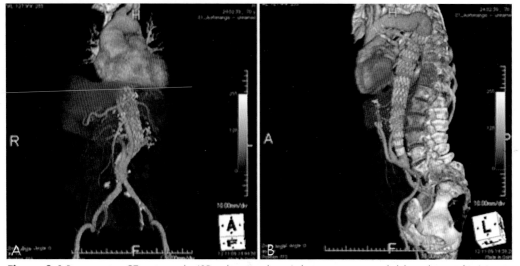

Figure 3.6 Postoperative CT-angiography (3D volume rendering) demonstrates visceral debranching with extraanatomic bypass grafting and endovascular aortic aneurysm repair (A: anterioposterioral axis, B: sagital axis).

The Viabahn open revascularization technique (VORTEC)

The Viabahn open revascularization technique (VORTEC) aims to avoid at least one anastomosis of the bypass branch with the target vessel, which is beneficial especially in case of demanding exposure and preparation of the target vessels.

The Viabahn stent-graft is introduced over a guidewire using the Seldinger technique via a puncture in the renal artery, SMA, or celiac trunk (Figure 3.7). After this the covered stent

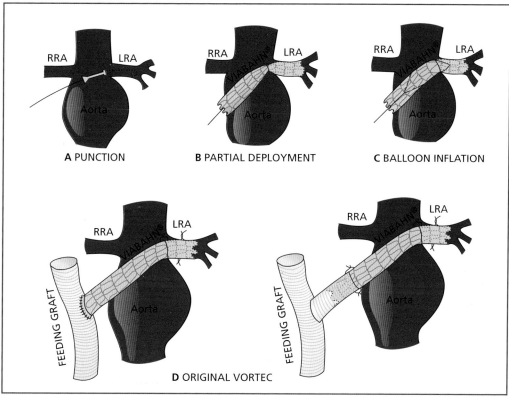

Figure 3.7 The several steps of the Viabahn open revascularization technique (VORTEC): punction of the left renal artery and introduction of the guide-wire in Seldinger technique in the renal artery. After this the covered stent is deployed partly within the artery and partly projecting outside the artery. Additionally the covered stent is dilated and two 6-0 polypropylene sutures are placed to fix the covered stent within the recipient artery. The proximal end of the stent-graft outside of the renal artery is sutured end to side directly to the main aortic graft or into the interposition graft. In the second, 6-0 prolene sutures are used for the Viabahn fixation to the graft.

is deployed partly within the artery and partly projecting outside the artery. Additionally the covered stent is dilated, and two 6-0 polypropylene sutures are placed to fix the covered stent within the recipient artery. The proximal end of the stent-graft outside of the renal artery is sutured end to side directly to the main aortic graft.

The technique was further developed through the use of an interposition branch graft on the main bypass graft and deployment of the proximal end of the stent-graft into the interposition branch graft. Additionally, the proximal end of the stent-graft are fixed with two 6-0 polypropylene sutures with the interposition branch graft avoiding another anastomosis. Finally, in the majority of the cases, the proximal stump of the target artery is ligated to avoid retrograde perfusion of the aneurysm.

Modified Viabahn open revascularization technique (mVORTEC)

The main benefit of the VORTEC is the avoidance of at least one anastomosis of the bypass branch with the target vessels. We modified the VORTEC for a high-risk patient with

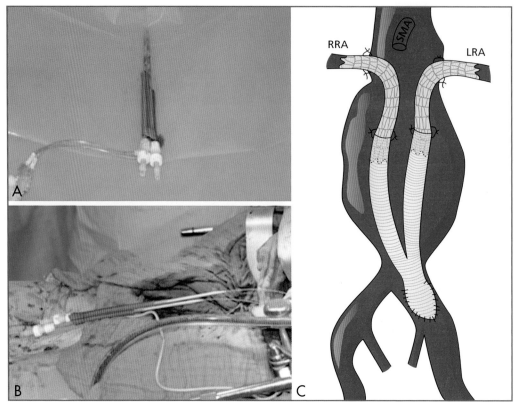

Figure 3.8 A) The two sheaths are preloaded into the two branches of the bifurcated graft. B) After punction of the renal arteries and insertion of the 0.035 Terumo wires in Seldinger technique the preloaded sheaths are going to be used for the insertion of the Viabahn stent-grafts. C) The sketch illustrates the modified viabahn open revascularization technique with deployment of the viabahns into the target vessels (renal arteries) and bypass branches. The proximal and distal parts of the Viabahns are fixed with 6-0 polypropylene sutures (no anastomoses are necessary).

PAAA with involvement of the renal arteries in the aneurysm. Two sheaths are preloaded in the branches of the bifurcated 14 mm Dacron bypass graft over 0.035 Terumo guide wires in order to advance and deploy Viabahn stent-grafts into the renals and into the branches of the bifurcated bypass (Figure 3.8 A,B). The proximal and distal part of the covered stents are fixed with two 6-0 polypropylene sutures. The final result is the avoidance of two anastomoses for each branch with deployment of the Viabahn into the renals and the bypass branches (Figure 3.8 C).

References

1. Black SA, Wolfe JH, Clark M. Complex thoracoabdominal aortic aneurysms: endovascular exclusion with visceral revascularization. J Vasc Surg 2006;43(6):1081-9.
2. Lachat M, Mayer D, Criado FJ, *et al.* New technique to facilitate renal revascularization with use of telescoping self-expanding stent grafts: VORTEC. Vascular 2008;16(2):69-72.
3. Kotsis T, Scharrer-Pamler R, Kapfer X, *et al.* Treatment of thoracoabdominal aortic aneurysms with a combined endovascular and surgical approach. Int Angiol 2003;22:125-33.

4. Fulton JJ, Farber MA, Marston WA, *et al.* Endovascular stent-graft repair of pararenal and type IV thoraco-abdominal aortic aneurysms with adjunctive visceral reconstruction. J Vasc Surg 2005;41:191-8.

5. Resch TA, Greenberg RK, Lyden SP, *et al.* Combined staged procedures for the treatment of thoracoabdominal aneurysms. J Endovasc Ther 2006;13:481-9.

6. Donas KP, Schulte S, Krause E, *et al.* Combined endovascular stent-graft repair and adjunctive visceral vessel reconstruction for complex thoracoabdominal aortic aneurysms. Int Angiol 2007;26:213-8.

7. Quinones-Baldrich W, Jimenez JC, DeRubertis B, *et al.* Combined endovascular and surgical approach (CESA) to thoracoabdominal aortic pathology: a 10-year experience. J Vasc Surg 2009;49:1125-34.

8. Biasi L, Ali T, Loosemore T, *et al.* Hybrid repair of complex thoracoabdominal aortic aneurysms using applied endovascular strategies combined with visceral and renal revascularization. J Thorac Cardiovasc Surg 2009;138:1331-8.

9. Donas KP, Lachat M, Rancic Z, *et al.* Early and midterm outcome of a novel technique to simplify the hybrid procedures in the treatment of thoracoabdominal and pararenal aortic aneurysms. J Vasc Surg 2009;50:1280-4.

10. Drinkwater SL, Böckler D, Eckstein H, *et al.* The visceral hybrid repair of thoraco-abdominal aortic aneurysms-a collaborative approach. Eur J Vasc Endovasc Surg 2009;38:578-85.

11. Kabbani LS, Criado E, Upchurch GR Jr, *et al.* Hybrid repair of aortic aneurysms involving the visceral and renal vessels. Ann Vasc Surg 2010;24:219-24.

12. Patel HJ, Upchurch GR Jr, Eliason JL, *et al.* Hybrid debranching with endovascular repair for thoracoabdominal aneurysms: a comparison with open repair. Ann Thorac Surg 2010;89:1475-81.

13. Chiesa R, Tshomba Y, Marone EM, *et al.* Hybrid procedures for the treatment of thoracoabdominal aortic aneurysms and dissections. J Cardiovasc Surg 2010;51:821-32.

14. Smith TA, Gatens S, Andres M, *et al.* Hybrid repair of thoracoabdominal aortic aneurysms involving the visceral vessels: comparative analysis between number of vessels reconstructed, conduit, and gender. Ann Vasc Surg 2011;25:64-70.

15. Schermerhorn ML, Giles KA, Hamdan AD, *et al.* Mesenteric revascularization: management and outcomes in the United States, 1988-2006. J Vasc Surg 2009;50:341-8.

16. Cherr GS, Hansen KJ, Craven TE, *et al.* Surgical management of atherosclerotic renovascular disease. J Vasc Surg 2002;35:236-45.

17. Lin P, Zhou W, Huynh T, *et al.* Hybrid repair of thoracoabdominal aortic aneurysm repair with visceral vessel debranching and aortic endograft exclusion: effect of staged versus simultaneous treatment approach on clinical outcomes. In: 32nd Annual Meeting of SAVS. January 16-19, 2008, Naples, FL.

CHAPTER 4

Planning fenestrated and branched endografts

M. Austermann, G. Torsello

The most crucial factor for successful endovascular treatment of complex aortic aneurysms is the exact planning of the endograft. The suggested planning of the physicians will be generally checked from the manufacturers who propose adjustments in order to get the best result especially in demanding anatomies.

For planning, a thin slice CT-scan (Figure 4.1) and modern software with the option of centerline reconstruction are essential. Because the endograft will straighten the anatomy, the

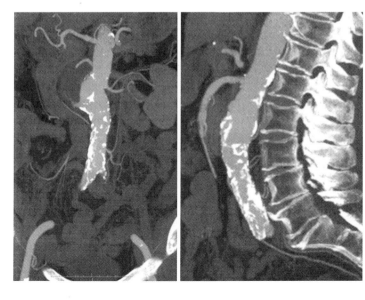

Figure 4.1 AP and lateral view of the abdominal aorta of a 82-year old female patient suffering from a suprarenal eccentric aortic aneurysm. The CT reconstruction of the aorta was performed using thin slice CT scan.

centerline should be corrected to a so called racing line. With this function it is possible to anticipate how the endograft will align in the aorta after deployment. Using the stretched reconstruction, the distances between the visceral arteries and renal arteries can be exactly measured and the clock position of the target vessels can be determined (Figures 4.2-4.4).

After obtaining an exact anatomical understanding of the aneurysm the next step will be to select a fenestrated or a branched endograft.

In juxtarenal aneurysms and some thoracoabdominal aneurysms the inner aortic diameter at the level of the visceral and renal arteries can be smaller than 30 mm. In such cases the use of a fenestrated graft is preferred (Figures 4.5-4.10). The fenestrated graft should have contact with the aortic wall at the level of the fenestrations in order to reduce the risk of type I or III endoleak. Pre-

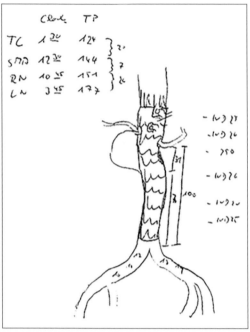

Figure 4.2 Preliminary drawing of the aneurysm with the most important measurements. Clock position of the fenestrations for the target vessels is determined.

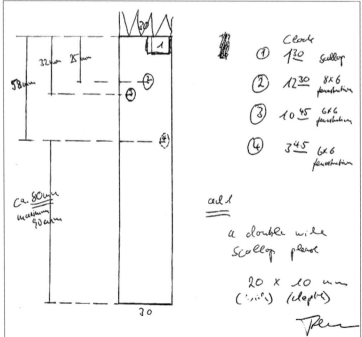

Figure 4.3 First sketch of the fenestrated graft, done by the physician.

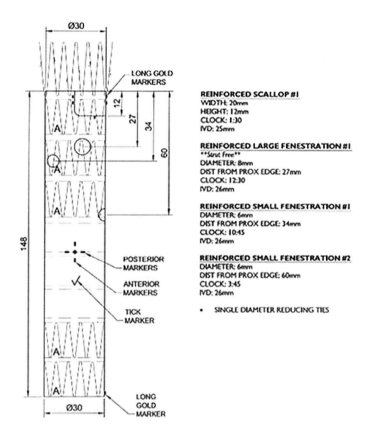

Ø30

LONG GOLD MARKERS

12
27
34
60

A

A

A

A

POSTERIOR MARKERS

ANTERIOR MARKERS

TICK MARKER

148

A

A

Ø30

LONG GOLD MARKER

REINFORCED SCALLOP #1
WIDTH: 20mm
HEIGHT: 12mm
CLOCK: 1:30
IVD: 25mm

REINFORCED LARGE FENESTRATION #1
Strut Free
DIAMETER: 8mm
DIST FROM PROX EDGE: 27mm
CLOCK: 12:30
IVD: 26mm

REINFORCED SMALL FENESTRATION #1
DIAMETER: 6mm
DIST FROM PROX EDGE: 34mm
CLOCK: 10:45
IVD: 26mm

REINFORCED SMALL FENESTRATION #2
DIAMETER: 6mm
DIST FROM PROX EDGE: 60mm
CLOCK: 3:45
IVD: 26mm

• SINGLE DIAMETER REDUCING TIES

Figure 4.4 Graft plan done by the planners of the manufacturing company.

cisely located fenestrations are crucial in order to avoid intraoperative problems probing the target vessels. Planning can be particularly demanding in difficult anatomies with kinking of the aorta at level of the fenestrations. In such cases it can be helpful to taper the graft down at the region of the fenestrations in order to have some gap between the fenestration and the ostia of the vessels. When the fenestration doesn't exactly match the vessel origin, this gap allows a possible cannulation of the target vessels. Covered stents are preferred as bridging devices, especially if there is no wall-opposition of the graft at this level. The stents should be long enough and accurately flared to achieve a good seal, avoiding type I or III endoleaks.

To achieve a stable position of the endograft at least two stent-rows should be in contact with healthy aortic wall. For treatment of juxtarenal aneurysms, 3 fenestrations and one scallop are typically required, while for suprarenal or thoracoabdominal aneurysms, 4 fenestrations are typically needed. The diameter of celiac trunk and SMA fenestrations is 8 mm in the majority of the patients and should be strut-free. The diameter of the renal artery fenestrations is usually 6×6 mm or 6×8 mm (Figures 4.2-4.4). All fenestrations should be secured by placement of covered stents. A preloaded catheter in one of the vessels (frequently the SMA) makes the access to the first fenestration easier. Through a small cut down of the axillary artery or of the cubital artery the access to the visceral vessels from above can be achieved easily, reducing the operation time.

In most cases, the fenestrated portion of the endograft is a tube and should be oversized

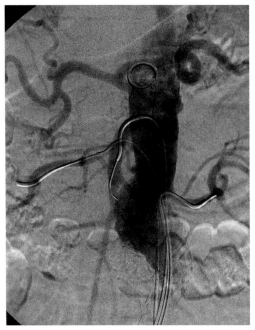

Figure 4.5 Angiography of the visceral aorta. Before introduction of the fenestrated graft target vessels are pre-cannulated with angiographic catheters.

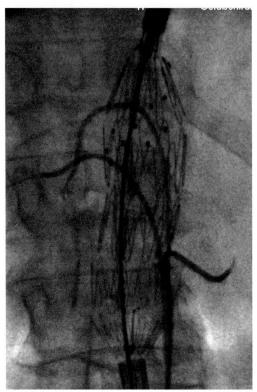

Figure 4.6 Exact placement of the fenestrated graft with the assistance of angiographic catheters placed into the visceral arteries.

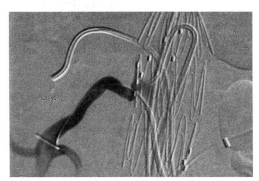

Figure 4.7 Cannulation of the right renal artery through the fenestration under guidance of the preplaced catheter.

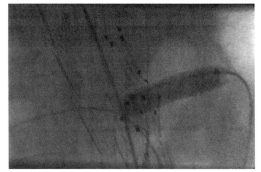

Figure 4.8 Stenting of the left renal artery with covered stent.

15-25% at the level of the sealing zone. The distal end of the graft should be 22 mm in diameter, so that an off the shelf bifurcated graft can be used as distal component. In case of thoracoabdominal aneurysms an additional thoracic graft is necessary. This graft is often tapered and should be implanted as a first step. The fenestrated graft should be 2 mm larger then the distal diameter of the thoracic endograft and should have an overlapping of at least 2, preferably 3 stent rows.

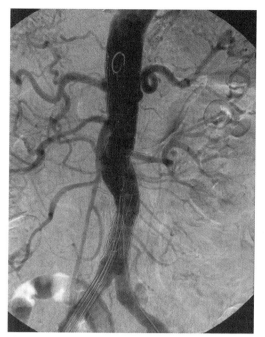

Figure 4.9 Completion angiography showing patent visceral vessels and no endoleak.

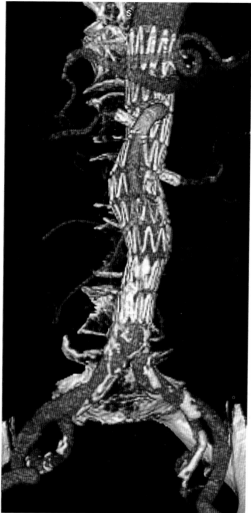

Figure 4.10 Follow-up CT scan showing complete exclusion of the aneurysm and patent visceral vessels.

In case of *thoracoabdominal aneurysms* with enough space at the level of the visceral and renal arteries (more than 30 mm) we prefer the use of endografts with cuffs (Figures 4.11-41.17). The overlapping between the bridging stent and the 18mm long branch gives the reconstruction more stability. Compared with the fenestrated graft, the cuffed endograft is much more forgiving in the planning.

The branches are usually 8 mm in diameter for the SMA and the celiac and 6 mm in diameter for the renal arteries. We mostly plan straight branches which opens about 10-20 mm above the related vessels (Figure 4.15). Helical branches are preferred when the target vessels have a tangential origin (Figures 4.18-4.24).

TIP: The first target vessel can be easily cannulated using a preloaded catheter for the SMA branch over a pull through wire.

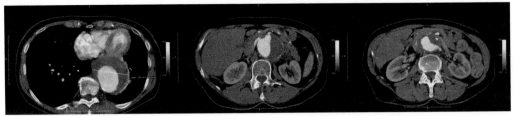

Figure 4.11 Thin slice CT-scan of a 70-year old female patient suffering from a thoracoabdominal aortic aneurysm with a diameter of 74 mm.

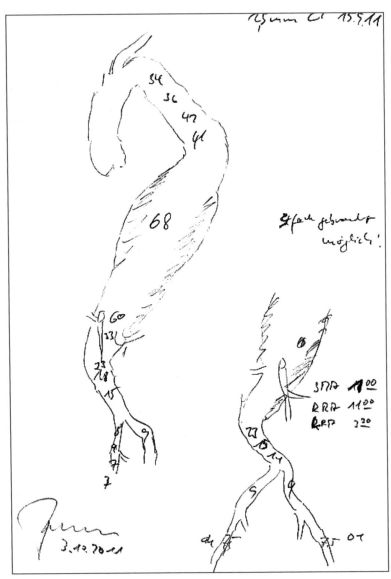

Figure 4.12 Sketch of the thoracoabdominal aneurysm with measurements of the most important diameters of the aorta and the clock position of the visceral arteries. Anatomical characteristics should be marked (done by the physician).

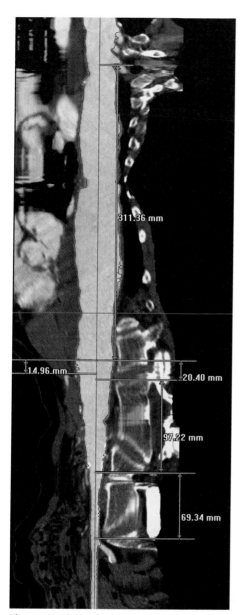

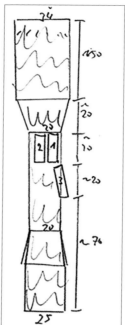

Figure 4.14 First drawing of the branched graft with three branches for SMA, RRA and LRA. The celiac trunk in this patient was completely occluded (done by the physician).

Figure 4.13 Stretched reconstruction of the TAAA with measurement of the distances between the visceral and renal arteries and between the left subclavian artery and the aortic bifurcation.

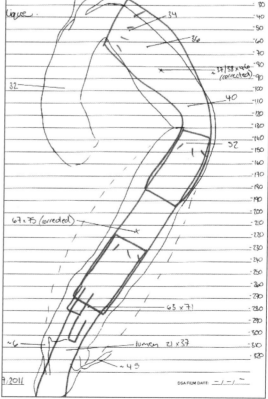

Figure 4.15 Anatomic sketch with planned endografts (done by the planners of the company after double checking).

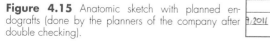

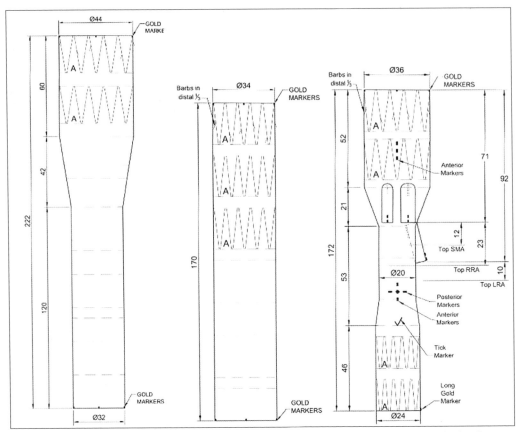

Figure 4.16 The final graft plan which has been done by the company must be approved and signed by the physician.

Using the so called trombone technique through a 12 F Flexor sheath (COOK), an 8 F Shuttle sheath can be advanced all the way down to the first branch. This enables stable positioning of the sheaths in the aorta. The introduction and advancement of catheters and stents is possible even through a demanding aortic arch or tortuous descending aorta.

The proximal diameter of the first thoracic endograft should be 15-25% oversized. Two, or preferably, three stent rows should be placed at the level of the proximal sealing zone. The thoracic endograft should end 4-5 cm above the celiac trunk, to have enough space for the first branch. The thoracic endograft has a distal diameter of 34 mm and the branched component starts with a diameter of 36 mm. Overlapping between the grafts should be three stent rows. If the space is not long enough for three stents, hooks can be used for fixation of the components. In this case, repositioning of the graft can be more difficult when the hooks contact the first graft. At the level of the branches the graft is tapered to have enough space for the cuffs and the bridging grafts. Usually, we taper the graft down to 22 mm in diameter. When the inner aortic diameter is below 30 mm it is possible to taper the graft down to 16 mm in diameter but excessive tapering can cause distal flow impairment.

The distal component of the endograft is usually a bifurcated graft, rarely a straight graft. The proximal diameter of this component is 24 mm providing adequate oversizing with the branched graft with a distal diameter of 22 mm.

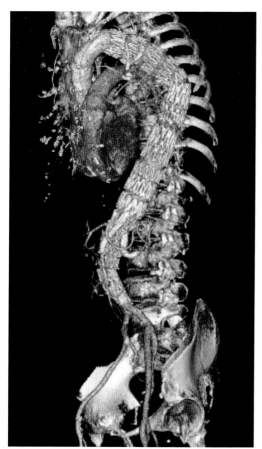

Figure 4.17 CT reconstruction after implantation of the brached endograft showing patent branches and no endoleak. Because of poor access vessels a 10 mm external conduit was previously implanted.

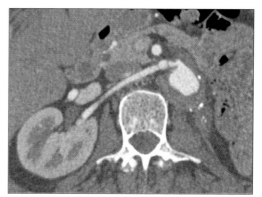

Figure 4.18 CT scan shows a tangential origin of the right renal artery.

Today, branched endografts are still customized and patient specific; however "off the shelf" devices will be available in the near future. The Cook T-branch device with 4 branches (Figure 4.25) will provide an off the shelf treatment option for TAAA. Also for fenestrated cases "off the shelf" endografts (Pivotal fenestrated device) are in the pipeline (Figure 4.26) and are being tested in controlled studies.

Planning in patients with aneurysm after thoracoabdominal dissection is particularly difficult. If the aneurysm involves the visceral portion of the aorta, aortic branches

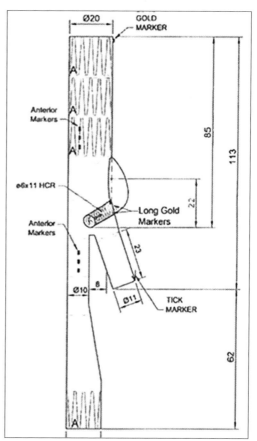

Figure 4.19 Helical branch for the RRA in order to have better access to this target vessel.

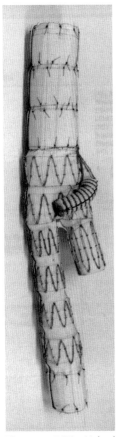

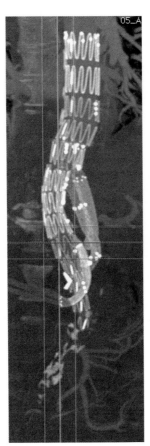

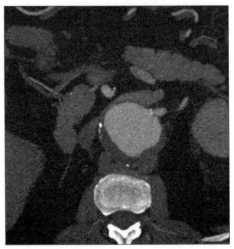

Figure 4.22 CT-scan of patient with aneurysm at level of the visceral aorta and solitary left kidney. Tangential origin of the left renal artery.

Figure 4.20 Helical branch for the right renal artery.

Figure 4.21 CT-scan after repair of the aneurysm with a branched graft. Note the helical branch for the RRA.

frequently originate from both the true and the false lumen. If the patients are at risk for open repair a complete endovascular approach with a fenestrated graft can be attempted after bright fenestration of the dissection lamella. Nevertheless, cannulation of the vessels remains demanding especially in patients with true lumen collapse or stenosis. In such cases a staged approach with treatment of the thoracic and thoracoabdominal aorta should be first performed to open and widen the true lumen. Planning of the fenestrated endograft should be done on the basis of a new CT scan.

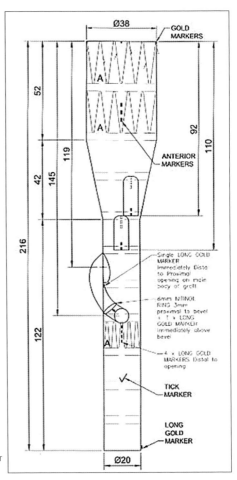

Figure 4.23 Graft plan of an endograft with two branches for the visceral arteries and helical branch for the left renal artery.

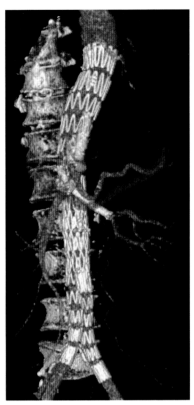

Figure 4.24 Postoperative CT scan showing good perfusion of all branches including the helical branch for the left renal artery.

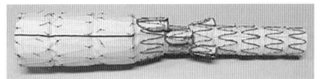

Figure 4.25 T-branch device.

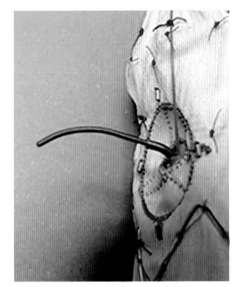

Figure 4.26 Pivotable fenestrated device.

CHAPTER 5

Use of fenestrated endografts

M. Austermann, G. Panuccio, G. Torsello

In complex aortic aneurysms, involvement of the aorta at the level of the renal and/or visceral branches may preclude stent-graft placement and sealing. New technologies such as fenestrated and branched grafts may create a suitable neck for adequate graft fixation. This technology was first suggested in the late 1990s and in 2005 received CE mark approval.

The most important indications for fenestrated grafts are:

- unsuitable proximal aneurysm neck for conventional EVAR;
- aneurysm with the renal artery originating from the distal portion of the aneurysm neck or accessory renal arteries with a diameter of >4 mm (Figure 5.1);
- aneurysm with involvement of the renal or visceral arteries;
- failure of previous open or endovascular aortic aneurysm repair with the proximal aneurysm involving the renal arteries.

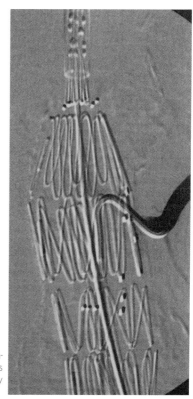

Figure 5.1 Fenestrated stent-graft for treatment of abdominal aortic aneurysm with involvement of an accessory renal artery. A SOS catheter has been used to pass through the single fenestration into the left accessory renal artery.

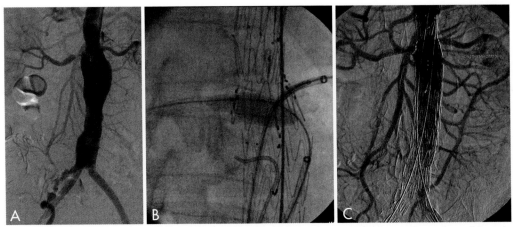

Figure 5.2 Angiography of a patient with aortic aneurysm involving the renal arteries (A). The stenosis of the right renal artery (B) represents a contraindication for fenestrated technique. Because of high risk profile of the patient for open surgery, endovascular treatment was performed. Through the fenestration the renal artery was dilated and stented as described below (C).

Not every patient is a good candidate for fenestrated technologies. The most important prerequisites are:
— catheterization of the iliac arteries is mandatory;
— aneurysm neck diameter should be below 42 mm;
— iliac diameter should range 8-22 mm;
— absence of severe aortic angulation;
— the renal and visceral arteries included in the graft should be >4 mm in diameter and free of severe stenosis. Only in high-risk patients for open surgery stenosis of target vessels can be treated before or during the aortic procedure (Figure 5.2);
— the implantation technique can be technically demanding. The operation should therefore be performed in angiosuites.

Fenestrated graft

The endografts consist of modular devices customized for individual patients; the geometric relationship of the target visceral vessels and the graft fenestrations are matched. The customization requires a high level of expertise to plan the graft and a few weeks for graft manufacturing and delivery. Planning, sizing and material knowledge are crucial for a good outcome (see chapter 4).

For the treatment of juxtarenal aortic aneurysms two major components are used. Depending on patient anatomy, additional ancillary products have to be customized.

The proximal component (Figure 5.3) is tubular in shape and contains all of the fenestrations. Three different types of fenestrations can be included in the proximal component to accommodate the anatomy of the visceral vessels:
— a scallop, usually positioned at the top of the stent-graft, which can have different sizes and may contain stent struts;
— small fenestrations measuring 4-6 mm in width and 4-8 mm in height are placed at the

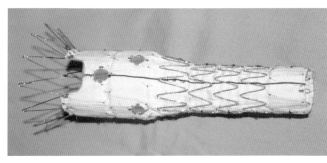

Figure 5.3 Proximal component of a fenestrated graft. The scallop is positioned at the top of the stent-graft and contains stent struts. Three small fenestrations for both renal arteries and for the superior mesenteric artery are placed at the primary site of seal. The fenestration for the SMA has a minimum distance of 15 mm from the fabric top. The small fenestrations do not include stent struts so that bridging stents can be introduced for sealing of the graft at this level.

primary site of seal with a minimum distance of 15 mm from the fabric top. They have an un-impended lumen as they do not include stent struts. Bare or covered stents are used for sealing at the level of the renal and visceral arteries;
– large fenestrations measuring 8-12 mm in diameter with a distance from the fabric top of 10 mm. They may contain crossing stent struts.

For better orientation, the proximal component contains a set of three markers vertically disposed in the anterior surface, and horizontally in the posterior surface (Figure 5.4), so that, after the deployment the markers form a cross in front (PA) view. By analogy with the Zenith Trifab graft an asymmetric "V" marker is also placed at the anterior side of the graft. Each fenestration also contains respectively 3 or 4 markers (Figure 5.5).

The release mechanism with the sequential knob has a gold release which withdraws the diameter reducing wire, a black one which detaches the proximal attachment and a white one which releases the distal attachment of the stent-graft (Figure 5.6). The distal diameter of the proximal component is usually 22 mm.

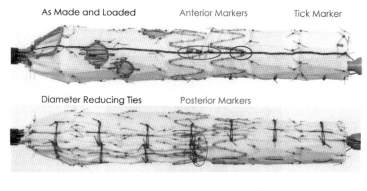

Figure 5.4 Anterior, posterior and tick markers help for better orientation and positioning of the endograft.

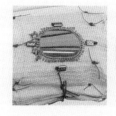
Reinforced Small Fenestration # 1 @ 10.00

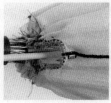
Reinforced Scallop # 1 @ 12.00

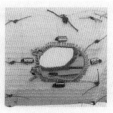
Reinforced Small Fenestration # 2 @ 2.30

Figure 5.5 Gold markers placed around the fenestration.

Control handle

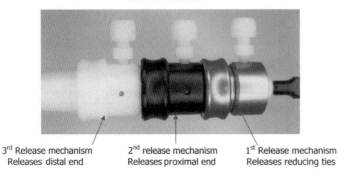

3rd Release mechanism
Releases distal end

2nd release mechanism
Releases proximal end

1st Release mechanism
Releases reducing ties

Figure 5.6 Sequential knob of the release mechanism. The gold release withdraws the diameter reducing wire, the black detaches the proximal attachment and the white releases the distal attachment of the stent-graft.

The distal component is usually bifurcated and has the trifab configuration of the Zenith device without a top bare stent. The proximal diameter is usually 24 mm.

Procedure

Vascular access

– Most fenestrated grafts require access through both femoral arteries. The ipsilateral is needed for the introduction of the main body, the contralateral is used for the access to the target vessels and for the contralateral leg. For this purpose, we use a 22 F Flexor sheath (Figure 5.7), which allows the simultaneous introduction of four sheaths for four different target vessels through the same sheath.
– At our institution most cases are performed with a complete percutaneous approach. In presence of a scar, severe calcification or aneurysm in the groin, cut down is mandatory.

TIP: resistance-free vascular accesses are mandatory to allow the fine-tune rotational and longitudinal movement of the graft to get the correct device position. In cases of small external

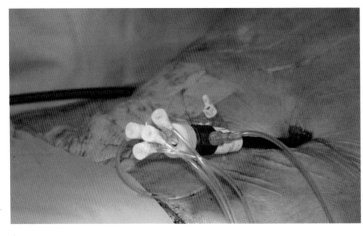

Figure 5.7 A 22 F Flexor sheath is introduced through a percutaneous contralateral femoral access. Up to four 5 F sheaths can be introduced through the valve and used for probing of the renal and visceral vessels using only one access.

iliac arteries, a common iliac artery approach through a conduit should be considered. Use of a dilatator (dotter angioplasty) or balloon and stents (cracking und paving method) has been also suggested as a bail out technique.

TIP: pre catheterization of the visceral vessels can be helpful to localize the origin of the visceral vessels and facilitate main body orientation. For this purpose a large introducer sheath (Extra Large Check-Flo® Introducers, Cook), between 18 F and 24 F, depending on the number of visceral vessels involved, is placed over a Lunderquist wire. The valve is punctured multiple times (accessory valve) and different 5 F sheaths can be advanced into the main sheath. Correct puncture of the valve and removal of the central guide wire are important to avoid bleeding from the sheath. Through the 5 F sheaths renal and visceral arteries are then cannulated with catheter-guidewire combination (SOS, SH or cobra) (Figures 5.8, 5.9).

TIP: recently, with the introduction of the fusion technique, the preoperative CT study can be matched with the patient position. The technique creates a roadmapping drawing virtual markers which reduces the amount of intraoperative contrast medium and fluoroscopy time.

Delivery and orientation of the proximal body

- Proper orientation of the proximal graft component is controlled by fluoroscopy using the gold markers (anterior, posterior and tick marker).
- The graft is then advanced over a Lunderquist wire under fluoroscopic visualization into the aorta until the fenestrations are just above the ostium of the respective target vessels. The outer sheath is withdrawn until the stent graft develops a diamond-like shape.

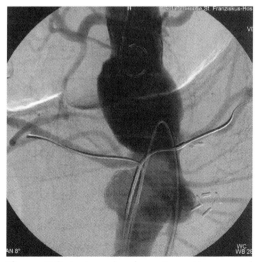

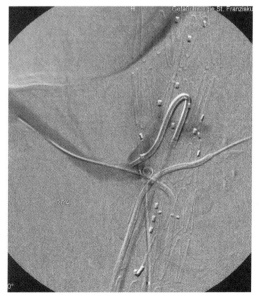

Figure 5.8 Angiography of a patient with suprarenal aortic aneurysm after previous open repair for infrarenal aneurysm. Demanding renal artery anatomy with calcification at the ostium. The origine of the right renal artery from the anterior aortic wall makes probing of the vessel difficult.

Figure 5.9 Precannulation of the renal artery facilitates both the orientation of the proximal fenestrated component and the access through the fenestration.

- After adjustment of the rotation, the sheath is completely withdrawn. Fine adjustments are still possible thanks to the diameter reducing ties. This is helpful especially in case the graft has to be derotated.

Bridge stent deployment

- The target vessel must be catheterized through the dedicated fenestration. For access to the target vessels, 7 F sheaths (usually 90 cm 7 F Shuttle sheath with high flex dilator 110 cm long, are used (Figure 5.10). The angiographic catheter has to match the patient anatomy. Double curved catheters (SOS, VS1, VS2) with soft wires are often used. Sometimes, it is necessary to first introduce the angiographic catheter into the aorta and then to pull it down into the renal artery.
- Once the catheter is in the target vessel, the soft guidewire is replaced with stiffer wires (Rosen, Cook or Supracore, Abbott).

TIP: in cases of difficult access the sheath can be advanced into the target vessels over PTA catheters during deflation of the PTA balloon.

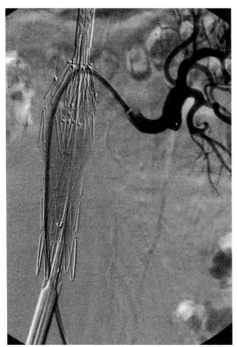

Figure 5.10 A 7 F sheath with a high flex dilator has been introduced through the fenestration into the left renal artery. Sometimes it is necessary to advance the sheath over a small balloon catheter which is first inflated at the ostium of the artery and then slowly deflated.

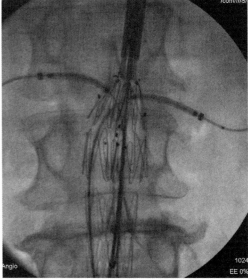

Figure 5.11 Through a 7 F sheath Advanta V12 covered stents (Atrium) are advanced into the renal arteries.

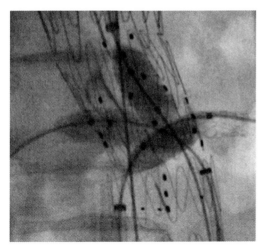

Figure 5.12 Using the tip of large balloon catheters (10x20 mm) the aortic portion of the covered stent is flared.

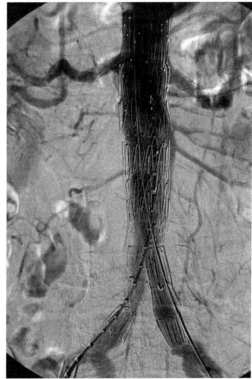

Figure 5.13 Completion angiography after aortic repair with a fenestrated stent-graft shows normal patency of the included target vessels without signs of endoleak.

- It can be very helpful to cannulate the SMA or the celiac trunk from a transbrachial access. In this case a preloaded catheter in the SMA fenestration is useful.
- The stents for the target vessels may then be advanced into the sheaths (Figure 5.11). Because of stent fractures observed after use of bare metal stents, covered stents (V12, Atrium) are now preferred. Bare metal stents are only used for small target vessels.
- The diameter reducing wires are then removed and the top cap deployed.
- After releasing the distal attachment the top cap is retrieved.
- The renal access sheaths are withdrawn and the renal stents are expanded.
- The aortic component of the renal stents should be flared (Figure 5.12) with the tip of a large PTA catheter (10-12 mm).
- After the proximal component sheath has been removed, the distal, usually bifurcated body is implanted in the usual manner. All the stent-graft components should have enough overlapping to avoid late type III endoleak.

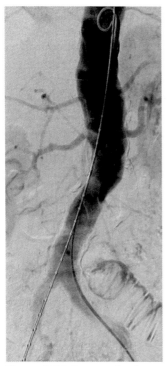

Figure 5.14 Angiography of a patient with a type IV aneurysm of the aorta. A 4-fenestrated endograft has been planned.

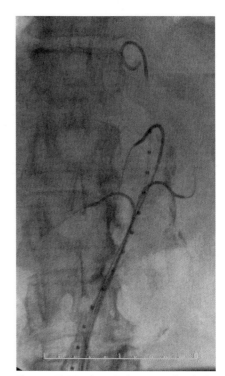

Figure 5.15 Through the same sheath the superior mesenteric artery and both renal arteries are precannulated with catheter wire combinations.

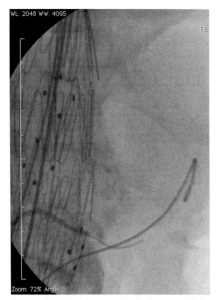

Figure 5.16 After partial deployment of the fenestrated component of the stent graft the left renal artery is cannulated through the dedicated fenestration.

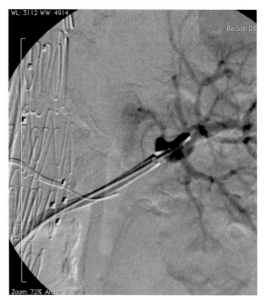

Figure 5.17 The correct position of the angiographic catheter and anatomy of the distal renal artery is checked by selective angiography. A Rosen wire is advanced through the catheter to give support to the 7 F sheath.

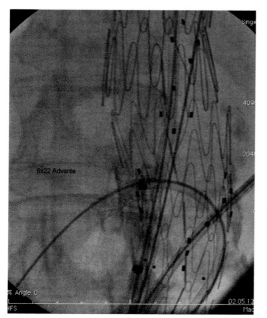

Figure 5.18 Over a 7 F sheath an Advanta covered stent is placed into both renal arteries.

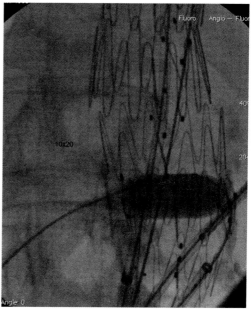

Figure 5.19 After deployment ob both renal stents flaring of the aortic portion is obtained with a large balloon catheter.

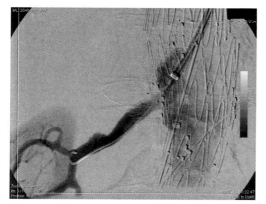

Figure 5.20 Selective angiography of the right renal artery showing good patency of the vessel and no signs of endoleak at this level.

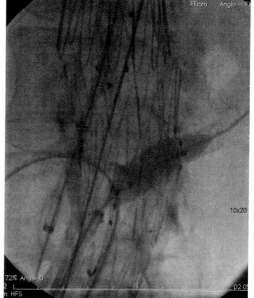

Figure 5.21 Flaring of the left renal stent.

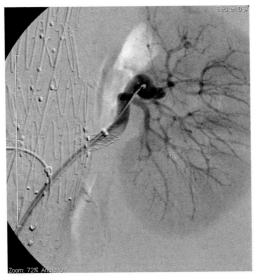

Figure 5.22 Selective angiography of the left renal artery after stenting.

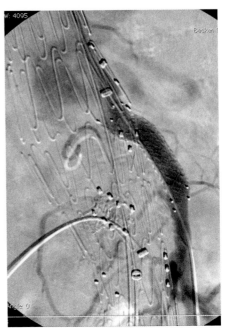

Figure 5.23 Selective angiography of the superior mesenteric artery. Cannulation of fenestration and vessel was performed through a left transbrachial approach. A long covered stent was used as bridging stent.

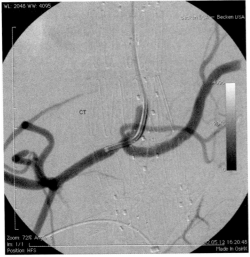

Figure 5.24 Angiography of the celiac trunk after passing the fenestration with a 5 F angiographic catheter.

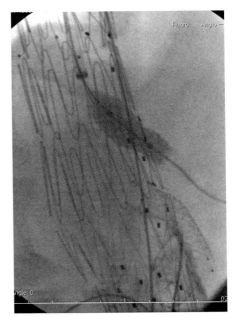

Figure 5.25 A large balloon expandable covered stent is deployed through the fenestration into the celiac artery.

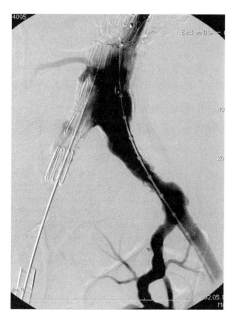

Figure 5.26 The bifurcated distal component of the stent graft has been deployed. A retrograde angiography through the sheath placed into the left EIA shows the left iliac bifurcation. A graduated catheter is used for the exact measurement of the left iliac limb.

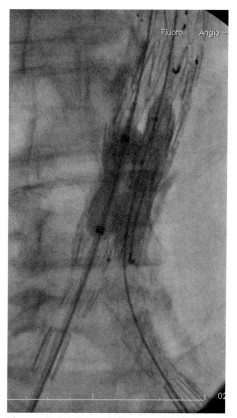

Figure 5.27 Kissing ballooning of both iliac arteries to avoid limb occlusion (narrow distal aortic diameter).

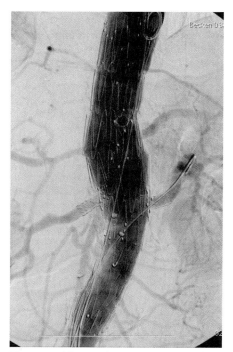

Figure 5.28 Completion angiography of the visceral aorta showing good patency of visceral and renal arteries and no endoleak.

– Completion angiography is performed to exclude endoleaks and document normal organ perfusion (Figure 5.13).

Figures 5.14-5.28 show step-by-step the implantation of a four-fenestrated stent graft.

References

1. Bakoyiannis CN, Economopoulos KP, Georgopoulos S, et al. Fenestrated and branched endografts for the treatment of thoracoabdominal aortic aneurysms: a systematic review. J Endovasc Ther 2010;17:201-9.
2. Greenberg RK, Sternbergh WC 3rd, et al. Fenestrated Investigators. Intermediate results of a United States multicenter trial of fenestrated endograft repair for juxtarenal abdominal aortic aneurysms. J Vasc Surg 2009;50(4):730-7.
3. Troisi N, Donas KP, Austermann M, et al. Secondary procedures after aortic aneurysm repair with fenestrated and branched endografts. J Endovasc Ther 2011;18:146-53.
4. Austermann M, Donas KP, Panuccio G, et al. Pararenal and thoracoabdominal aortic aneurysm repair with fenestrated and branched endografts: lessons learned and future directions. J Endovasc Ther 2011;18:157-60.
5. Torsello GB, Kasprzak B, Klenk E, et al. Endovascular suture versus cutdown for endovascular aneurysm repair: a prospective randomized pilot study. J Vasc Surg 2003;38:78-82.
6. Amiot S, Haulon S, Becquemin JP, et al. Fenestrated endovascular grafting: the French multicentre experience. Eur J Vasc Endovasc Surg 2010;39:537-44.
7. Greenberg RK, Sternbergh WC, Makaroun M, et al. Intermediate results of a United States multicenter trial of fenestrated endograft repair for juxtarenal abdominal aortic aneurysms. J Vasc Surg 2009;50:730-7.
8. Dowdall JF, Greenberg RK, West K, et al. Separation of components in fenestrated and branched endovascular grafting - branch protection or a potentially new mode of failure? Eur J Vasc Endovasc Surg 2008;36:2-9.
9. O'Neill S, Greenberg RK, Haddad F, et al. Prospective analysis of fenestrated endovascular grafting: intermediate-term outcomes. Eur J Vasc Endovasc Surg 2006;32:115-23.
10. Sun Z, Mwipatayi BP, Semmens JB, et al. Short to midterm outcomes of fenestrated endovascular grafts in the treatment of abdominal aortic aneurysms: a systematic review. J Endovasc Ther 2006;13:747-53.
11. Semmens JB, Lawrence-Brown MM, Hartley DE, et al. Outcomes of fenestrated endografts in the treatment of abdominal aortic aneurysm in Western Australia (1997-2004). J Endovasc Ther 2006;13:320-9.
12. Patterson BO, Hinchliffe RJ, Holt PJ, et al. Importance of aortic morphology in planning aortic interventions. J Endovasc Ther 2010;17:73-7.

CHAPTER 6

Use of branched endografts for thoracoabdominal aneurysms

M. Austermann, G. Torsello

As open surgery for thoracoabdominal aortic aneurysm (TAAA) is associated with high morbidity and mortality rates, endovascular techniques with branched technology have been developed during the last years.

The most important clinical and anatomic indications for use of branched grafts in patients with TAAA are:
– TAAA with a diameter of ≥6 cm or with rapid expansion;
– suitable anatomy for endovascular repair which includes:
  • catheterization of the arch through the brachial vessels must be possible;
  • aneurysm neck diameter <42 mm;
  • iliac diameter should be at least 8 mm. If iliac arteries have a smaller diameter, implantation of an external conduit should be performed (Figure 6.1);
  • aortic angulation should be below 80° unless through-and-through

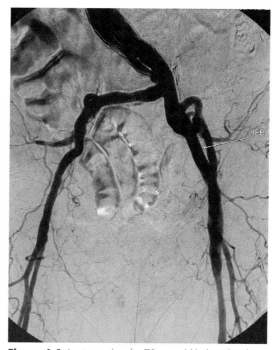

Figure 6.1 Angiography of a 78-year old lady with a thoracoabdominal aneurysm and tortuousity of the left iliac artery. A bypass graft between the left common iliac and the left superficial femoral artery has been previously implanted to be used as external conduit.

wires and ballooning can help to advance the stent grafts through severe angulated anatomy (Figure 6.2);

- the diameter of the arteries included in the graft should be >4 mm and the cannulation must be possible;
- the inner aortic diameter should be at least 25 mm, providing enough space for the branches.

The anatomic limitations of these technologies are:
- presence of a small true lumen in case of aneurysm after dissection;
- aortoiliac anatomy which impairs trackability of large bore sheaths;
- non-availability of off-the-shelf devices for emergent situations. The introduction of the T-branch device will enable the treatment of a greater number of patients in the next future (see chapter 4).

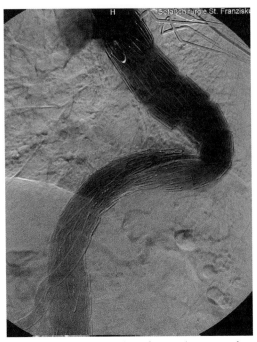

Figure 6.2 Angiography after implantation of a branched stent-graft for thoracoabdominal aneurysm. Aortic angulation >80° is usually a contraindication. In this patients who did not have other surgical options staged procedure was performed. As first step a thoracic endograft was implanted. As trackability of the graft through the angulated anatomy during the first endografting was possible, a branched stent-graft was used in a second step for repairing of the thoracoabdominal aorta.

Endograft

The thoracoabdominal aorta is primarily treated with a branch-bearing stent graft manufactured by Cook (Figure 6.3). The graft has a wide proximal and distal segment with a narrow segment in the middle containing the cuffs. The distal diameter of the graft is usually 22 mm. The branch bearing segment can be down tapered to 16 mm. Because of potential hemodynamic issues, lower diameters should be exceptionally used. A variable number of cuffs is usually caudally oriented and positioned to correspond to the branches which have to be included. The cuffs are usually 6-8 mm in diameter and 18-22 mm in length.

The endograft is provided with markers indicating the proximal and distal end of each cuff (Figure 6.4).

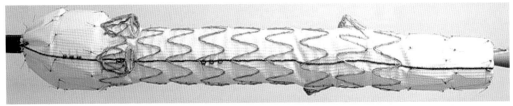

Figure 6.3 The primary component of the thoracoabdominal side-branch endovascular graft is a cuff-bearing stent graft with a wide proximal and distal segment and with a narrow segment in the middle containing the cuffs. In this case two cuffs for the visceral arteries are oriented caudally and two (for the renal arteries) are oriented cranially.

Additional components as proximal extensions (standard Zenith TX-2) and distal extensions (modified Zenith bifurcated stent graft) are respectively used in cases of thoracic or/and abdominal involvement of the aneurysm. In patients with extended thoracoabdominal aneurysms, a staged procedure with implantation of the proximal thoracic extension can be useful to reduce the risk of paraplegia.

Procedure

– Access
  • Most branched grafts for TAAA require access through both femoral arteries and the subclavian artery. Depending on the number of branches, cut down of the axillary or of the subclavian artery may be necessary.
  • Femoral access is needed for the introduction of the primary component and of the extensions. The use of a surgical conduit with a 10 mm graft can facilitate access in patients with a challenging iliac anatomy (Figure 6.1).
  • In case of type II and III TAAA (Figure 6.5) the proximal, and in most cases tapered, extension is deployed at the level of the descending thoracic aorta, avoiding overstenting of the left subclavian artery for the access to the target vessels.
– Orientation
  • Previously placed catheters and wires into the visceral and renal arteries facilitate orientation and cannulation of the target vessels through the fenestrations (Figure 6.6).
  • The correct orientation of the primary graft component is then checked by fluoroscopy (Figure 6.7). Three anterior/posterior markers and the tick marker help to find the right clock position of the branched component.
– Deployment of the main body
  • Over a stiff wire (Lunderqvist, Cook) the cuff-bearing graft is advanced into the aorta and placed with the branches 10-20 mm above the orifice of the respective target vessels. The position of the cuffs has been oriented to the circumferential position of the visceral arteries beforehand.
  • The graft is deployed by withdrawing the outer sheath and pulling the control wires.
– Deployment of the branches
  • 7 F or 8 F sheaths (usually 90 cm long Shuttle sheaths with a 110 cm long high flex dilator) are advanced through a 12 F Flexor sheath in order to acquire access to the target vessels. Using a catheter-guide wire combination (vertebral or multipurpose catheter

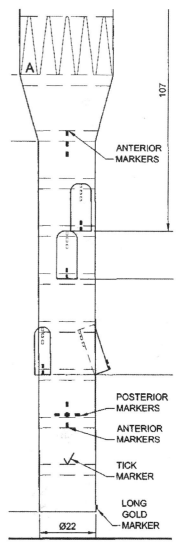

Figure 6.4 The endograft is provided with markers indicating the proximal and distal end of each cuff and similarly to the fenestrated with anterior and posterior markers.

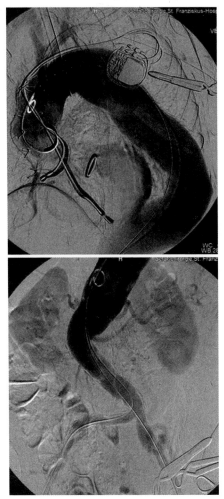

Figure 6.5 Angiography of a patient with a type III thoracoabdominal aortic aneurysm.

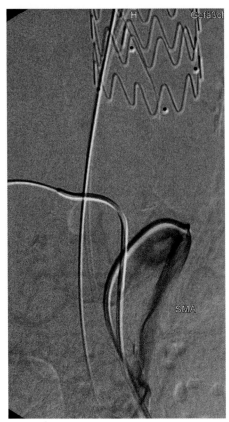

Figure 6.6 The thoracic extension has been implanted in the descending aorta with the distal end 3 cm above the origin of the celiac trunk. The origin of the visceral arteries are marked with angiographic catheters.

with soft wires), an access to the target vessels can then be obtained (Figure 6.8). To get access through the first branch while the graft is still proximally and distally fixed, a preloaded catheter in one of the branches can be helpful.

- After replacing the soft guidewire for a stiffer wire (Rosen wire, Cook), the 7 F or 8 F sheath is advanced into the target vessels (Figure 6.9).
- Covered stents are then advanced and deployed (Figures 6.10-6.12). Depending on the length of the segment which has to be covered and the need for flexibility, different covered stents (V12, Atrium, Viabahn, Gore or Fluency, Bard) are used (Figure 6.13). The overlapping between covered stent and target vessel is usually 10-20 mm and between the covered stent and the cuff 20-25 mm. Only in case of early bifurcated target vessel a shorter overlapping can be accepted. Relining with an oversized bare stent is often required (Figure 6.10).

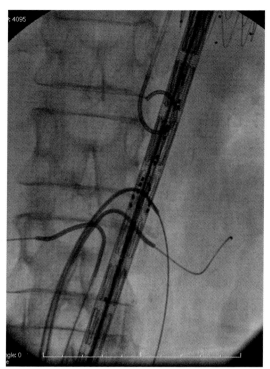

Figure 6.7 The cuff-bearing graft is advanced into the aorta and placed with the branches 10-20 mm above the orifice of the respective target vessel. The position of the cuffs is oriented to the circumferential position of the visceral arteries. The previously placed catheters and wires into the visceral and renal arteries facilitate the orientation.

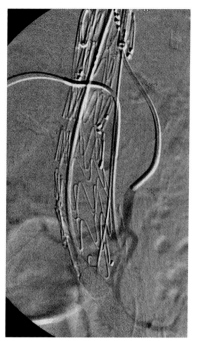

Figure 6.8 After deployment of the graft a 8F sheath is advanced into the cuff. The access to the SMA is obtained with a catheter-guide wire combination.

– Procedure completion

• If the abdominal aorta is involved, a distal, usually bifurcated graft has to be implanted (Figure 6.14). All components have to be deployed with enough overlapping to avoid late type III endoleak.

• Completion angiography is performed to exclude endoleaks and document normal organ perfusion (Figure 6.15).

• In patients at high-risk for paraplegia (extended coverage of the aorta) CSF pressure has to be carefully monitored and corrected.

• Figures 6.16-6.29 show the procedure step-by-step.

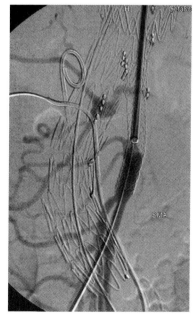

Figure 6.9 The soft guidewire is replaced with a stiffer wire and the 8F sheath is advanced into the SMA. A covered stent can now be deployed without covering important branches of the SMA.

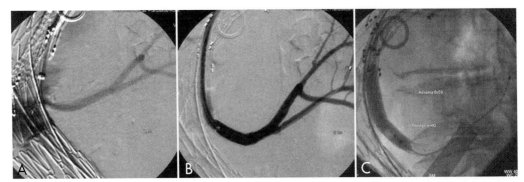

Figure 6.10 The angiography (A) shows an angulated and severe calcified origin of the left renal artery. The combination (B) of a high radial force covered stent (Advanta V12, Atrium) and a flexible self-expandable bare stent increases kinking resistance of the bridging stent (C).

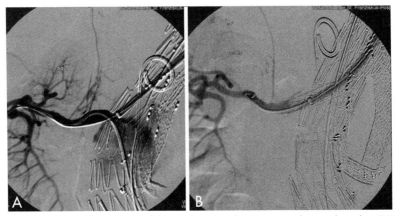

Figure 6.11 The cannulation of the renal artery with a Rosen guide wire through a 7 F sheath (A) and the implantation of the covered stent is on the right side easier to perform (B).

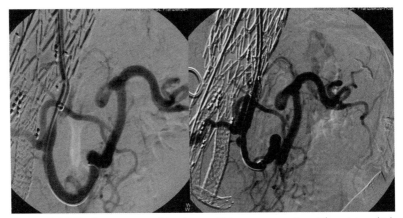

Figure 6.12 The last target vessel (coeliac trunk) shows a narrowing at the origin, which can be passed with a soft guidewire catheter combination. Also in this case an Advanta covered stent is used as a bridging stent.

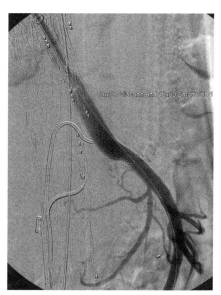

Figure 6.13 When the distance between cuff and target vessel is longer than 5 cm a self-expanding covered stent (Viabahn, Gore or Fluency, Bard) should be used. An overlapping between covered stent and target vessel of 20 mm and between the covered stent and the cuff of 20-25 mm is recommended.

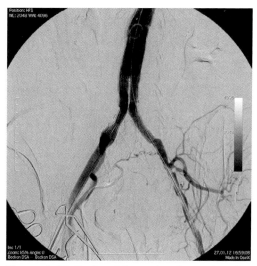

Figure 6.14 Finally a bifurcated graft is implanted to treat the infrarenal portion of the aneurysm. All the components have to be deployed with enough overlapping to avoid late type III endoleak.

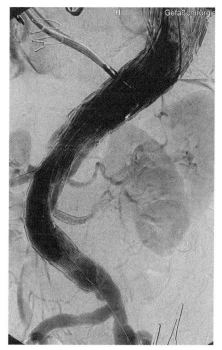

Figure 6.15 Completion aortography showing the patency of the target vessels.

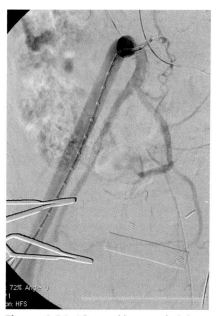

Figure 6.16 65-year old man with 8.9 cm aneurysm of the thoracoabdominal aorta with stenosis of the access vessels. Retrograde angiography through the right groin showing surgical conduit (10 mm Dacron graft) between the right common iliac artery and the right femoral artery. The conduit was necessary because of the diffuse stenotic lesion of the external iliac artery.

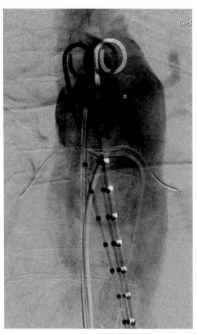

Figure 6.17 Aortography showing both renal arteries coming from the partially thrombosed aortic aneurysm. To facilitate orientation and cannullation of the branches in this demanding anatomy precannulation with angiographic catheters is performed.

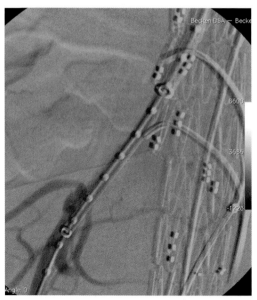

Figure 6.18 The superior mesenteric artery has been cannulated with a 8F sheath. A selective angiography shows the branches of the SMA. Using a graduated angiographic catheter the optimal length of the stent can be determined.

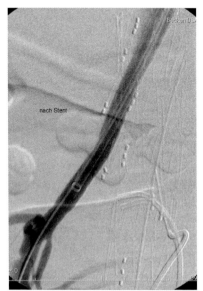

Figure 6.19 Selective angiography of the SMA after implantation of a 7x59 mm Advanta covered stent. The stent was postdilated with an 8 mm PTA catheter.

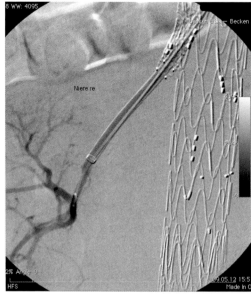

Figure 6.20 Selective angiography of the right renal artery showing diseased renal branches.

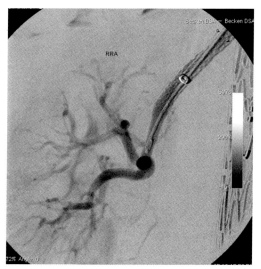

Figure 6.21 Angiography after placement of balloon expandable covered stent into the right renal artery.

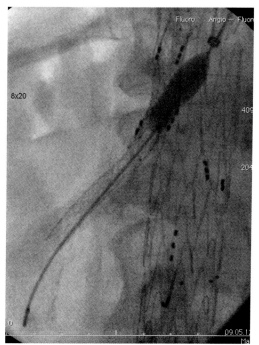

Figure 6.22 Flaring of the proximal portion of the renal stent.

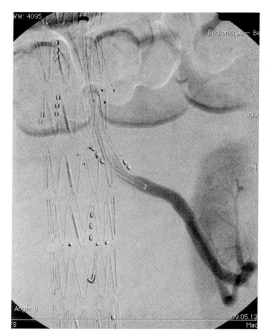

Figure 6.23 Selective angiography of the left renal artery after stenting as described for the right side.

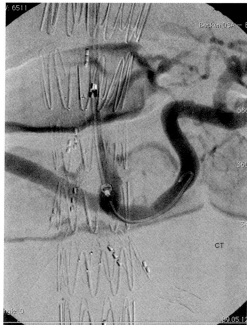

Figure 6.24 Through a transaxillary approach the celiac artery has been easily cannulated. The selective angiography shows the origin of the branches.

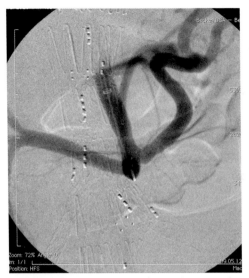

Figure 6.25 Angiography after implantation of a 8x39 Advanta covered stent.

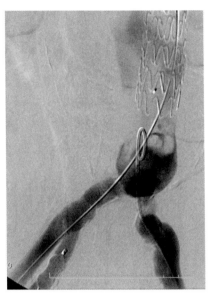

Figure 6.26 Angiography showing the aortic bifurcation and the conduit on the right side. The right common iliac artery is short. To avoid distal type I endoleak coil occlusion of the distal common iliac artery below the anastomosis artery has been performed using an Amplatzer device. With this technique retrograde perfusion of the hypogastric artery remained possible.

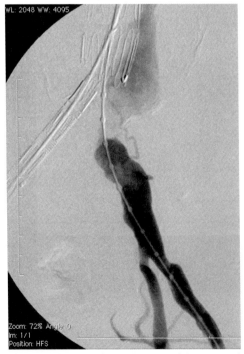

Figure 6.27 The bifurcated portion of the stent graft has been partially deployed. The contralateral gate has been cannulated. Retrograde angiography of the left iliac vessels shows the origin of the left hypogastric artery, which has to be preserved. The graduated angiographic catheter left in place helps by measuring the length of the contralateral iliac limb.

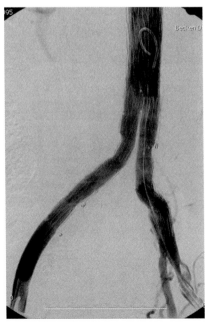

Figure 6.28 Angiography of the bifurcated component of the endograft.

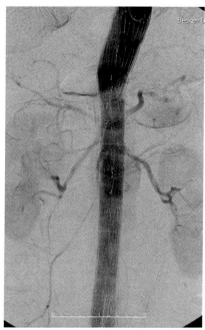

Figure 6.29 Completion angiography showing the proximal cuffed component of the endograft and the good patency of branches and target vessels.

References

1. Reilly LM, Chuter TA. Endovascular repair of thoracoabdominal aneurysms: design options, device construct, patient selection and complications. J Cardiovasc Surg 2009;50:447-60.
2. Eagleton MJ, Greenberg RK. Late complications after endovascular thoracoabdominal aneurysm repair. Semin Vasc Surg 2009;22:87-92.
3. Chuter TA, Hiramoto JS, Park KH, *et al.* The transition from custom-made to standardized multibranched thoracoabdominal aortic stent grafts. J Vasc Surg 2011;54:660-8.
4. Cowan JA Jr, Dimick JB, Henke PK, *et al.* Surgical treatment of intact thoracoabdominal aortic aneurysms in the United States: hospital and surgeon volume-related outcomes. J Vasc Surg 2003;37:1169-74.
5. Chuter TA, Gordon RL, Reilly LM, *et al.* Multi-branched stent-graft for type III thoracoabdominal aortic aneurysm. J Vasc Interv Radiol 2001;12:391-2.
6. Anderson JL, Adam DJ, Berce M, *et al.* Repair of thoracoabdominal aortic aneurysms with fenestrated and branched endovascular stent grafts. J Vasc Surg 2005;42:600-7.
7. Greenberg RK, Lytle B. Endovascular repair of thoracoabdominal aneurysms. Circulation 2008;117: 2288-96.
8. Muhs BE, Verhoeven EL, Zeebregts CJ, *et al.* Mid-term results of endovascular aneurysm repair with branched and fenestrated endografts. J Vasc Surg 2006;44:9-15.
9. Roselli EE, Greenberg RK, Pfaff K, *et al.* Endovascular treatment of thoracoabdominal aortic aneurysms. J Thorac Cardiovasc Surg 2007;133:1474-82.
10. Chuter TA, Rapp JH, Hiramoto JS, *et al.* Endovascular treatment of thoracoabdominal aortic aneurysms. J Vasc Surg 2008;47:6-16.
11. Bakoyiannis CN, Economopoulos KP, Georgopoulos S, *et al.* Fenestrated and branched endografts for the treatment of thoracoabdominal aortic aneurysms: a systematic review. J Endovasc Ther 2010;17:201-9.
12. Verhoeven EL, Tielliu IF, Bos WT, *et al.* Present and future of branched stent grafts in thoraco-abdominal aortic aneurysm repair: a single-centre experience. Eur J Vasc Endovasc Surg 2009;38:155-61.

CHAPTER 7

Use of iliac side branch devices for aortoiliac aneurysms

G. Torsello, M. Austermann

Among patients with AAA, 20% also have aneurysmal iliac arteries. The location of the iliac arteries makes open repair challenging, especially in obese and high-risk patients. Endovascular repair with hypogastric occlusion has been proposed as a less-invasive alternative, but one third of patients treated in this manner develop severe buttock claudication after coiling of the internal iliac artery. The use of iliac side branch devices (IBD) can preserve pelvic flow, and decreases the risk of buttock claudication, erectile dysfunction and bowel ischemia in patients with AAA involving the iliac artery.

The most important anatomic indication and prerequisites for the use of iliac side branched endografts are:

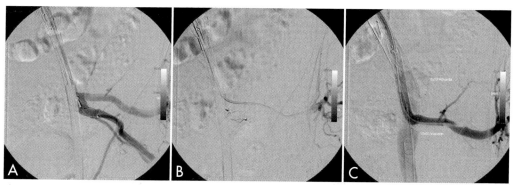

Figure 7.1 Angiography of a patient with aortoiliac aneurysm without adequate landing zone at level of the distal internal iliac artery (A). After coil embolization of one branch of the IIA (B) the distal end of the bridging stent can be placed more distally preserving the gluteal perfusion (C). The distal fixation zone of the bridging stent reduces the risk of stent migration and type I or II endoleak.

- common iliac artery (CIA) aneurysm with diameter >26 mm and length >50 mm;
- patent CIA lumen >18 mm;
- iliac artery bifurcation diameter > 15 mm;
- adequate length of the external iliac artery (EIA) for a distal landing zone of > 20 mm;
- diameter of external iliac artery between 8 mm and 18 mm;
- sufficient long landing zone (>10 mm) at the internal iliac artery (IIA);
- diameter of the IIA at the landing zone <11 mm.

HINT: In high-risk patients a distal landing zone can be created by coil embolization of one branch of the IIA (Figure 7.1).

Zenith Branch Endovascular Graft-Iliac Bifurcation

For the treatment of iliac artery aneurysms, the Zenith Branch™ Endovascular Graft-Iliac Bifurcation (Cook) is used (Figure 7.2), typically in conjunction with a covered stent. The device, which is CE-marked since August 2006, is a bifurcated branch vessel graft with openings to connect the common iliac, internal iliac side branch, and external iliac segments. The delivery system has a preloaded indwelling catheter to facilitate cannulation of the side branch.

The endograft has four radiopaque gold markers to facilitate fluoroscopic visualization and orientation of the stent graft. The markers are positioned along the internal iliac side of the proximal portion of the graft to indicate the position of the side branch segment (Figure 7.3). The indwelling catheter and markers are aligned with the most lateral aspect of the side branch. The second marker from the distal end (2D) is the target marker for the most proximal location of the proximal end of the covered stent that is used to extend the side branch into the internal iliac artery. The second marker from the proximal end (2P) is the target

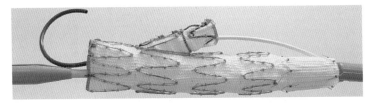

Figure 7.2 The Zenith Branch Endovascular Graft-Iliac Bifurcation is a bifurcated branch vessel graft with a preloaded indwelling catheter to facilitate cannulation of the side branch.

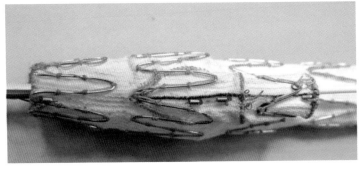

Figure 7.3 Four radiopaque gold markers indicate the position of the sidebranch segment. The second marker from the distal end indicates the most proximal location of the proximal end of the bridging covered stent. The second marker from the proximal end indicates the most distal location of the distal end of the leg extension that will connect the iliac side branch to the bifurcated aortic stent graft.

marker for the most distal location of the distal end of the leg extension. The leg extension connects the iliac side branch with the bifurcated stent graft, which is deployed above the aortic bifurcation.

Isolated aneurysms of the CIA can be treated with this device. But usually, a Zenith AAA graft is additionally needed because of inadequate neck at level of the CIA or involvement of the aorta.

The contralateral iliac artery is treated with a conventional iliac leg if the diameter is <26 mm or with an IBD in case of contralateral CIA aneurysm.

Procedure

- Access through both femoral arteries either by percutaneous technique or cut-down. In patients with previous implanted aortic bifurcated graft an additional transbrachial approach is needed (Figure 7.4).
- The target internal iliac artery should be imaged prior to deploying an IBD. Oblique projections are required for identification of the origin of the hypogastric artery (Figure 7.5).
- After fluoroscopic orientation of the side branch segment, the Zenith Bifurcated Iliac Side Branch device is introduced over a stiff wire through the side of the common iliac artery

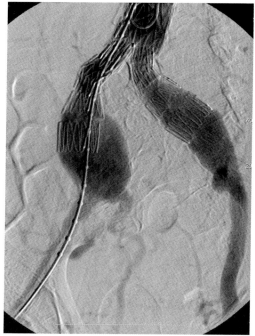

Figure 7.4 Angiography of a patient previously treated with a bifurcated aortic graft. The patient developed an aneurysm of both common iliac arteries with involvement of the iliac bifurcation. For treatment with an IBD, transbrachial access for the placement of the bridging stents is additionally needed.

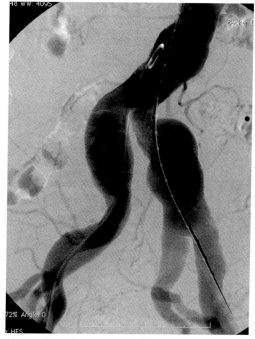

Figure 7.5 Angiography with oblique projection is needed for identification of the origin of the left hypogastric artery.

aneurysm to be treated. The device is inserted until the tip of the indwelling catheter is just above the aortic bifurcation.

– After partial deployment of the device, the curved tip of the preloaded catheter is visible and a stiff hydrophilic guide wire is advanced and snared through a contralateral approach with a goose neck catheter or an Indy Snare (Cook).

– The device is deployed until the distal end of the side branch is exposed and positioned 10-20 mm above the origin of the internal iliac artery.

– A 12F Flexor sheath is advanced over the through-and-through wire guide until it enters the side branch. To facilitate the maneuver, remove the preloaded catheter and clamp the hydrophilic through-and-through wire guide at both ends and pull on both sides (Figure 7.6).

– The IIA is catheterized with a vertebral or multipurpose angiographic catheter (Figure 7.7) through a separate puncture of the valve of the 12 F sheath. The soft guide wire is changed for a stiffer wire (*e.g.*, Rosen) and the angiographic catheter is removed.

– A bridging covered stent is advanced through a 7 F sheath and deployed with respect to the side branch overlap (10-14 mm) and the intended internal iliac artery fixation site.

– HINT: Caution must be taken when advancing balloon-expandable stents. Preloading of the covered stent in the 7 F sheath can be helpful. Different oblique projections (in comparison to those needed to identify the origin of the hypogastric artery) are required for identification of the distal landing zone.

– Depending on the distance that has to be covered and the need for flexibility, different

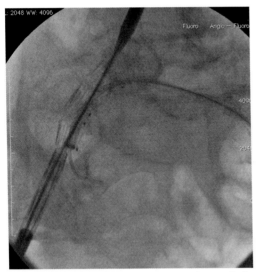

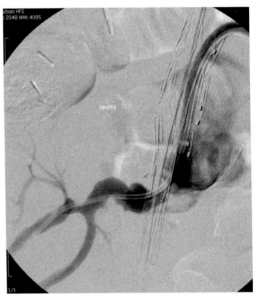

Figure 7.6 The Zenith Bifurcated Iliac Side Branch device is introduced through the side of the common iliac artery aneurysm to be treated. The device was deployed until the distal end of the side branch was exposed and positioned 10 mm above the origin of the internal iliac artery. Over a through-and-through wire guide a 12F sheath is advanced until it enters the main body and the side branch.

Figure 7.7 The IIA is catheterized with a soft angiographic catheter-guide wire combination. The soft guide wire is changed for a stiffer wire (Rosen) and the catheter removed. For identification of the distal landing zone a different oblique projection is required than for identification of the origin of the hypogastric artery.

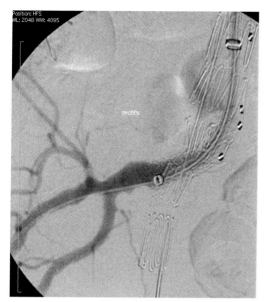

Figure 7.8 Through a 7 F sheath a bridging covered stent is advanced and deployed with respect to the side branch overlap and the hypogastric artery. For better wall apposition of the balloon expandable covered stent flaring with a larger balloon can be performed. Relining with an oversized self-expanding bare stent is sometimes required.

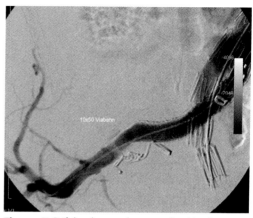

Figure 7.9 If the distance between distal landing zone and the IBD is longer than 5 cm, a flexible self-expandable covered stent (Viabahn or Fluency) is preferred. The overlapping between covered stent and target vessel should be at least 10-20 mm. Coil embolization of the first branch was performed because of a short landing zone at level of the IIA.

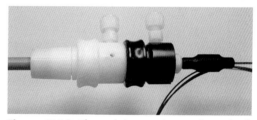

Figure 7.10 After withdrawing the introducer sheath of the graft until the external iliac component is fully deployed, the safety lock and the black trigger-wire release mechanism must be removed. Then withdraw and remove the white trigger-wire by sliding the white trigger-wire release mechanism.

covered stents (*e.g.*, V12, Atrium, NH or Viabahn, Gore, Fluency, Bard) are used (Figures 7.8, 7.9).
- The overlap between the covered stent and target vessel is usually 10-20 mm and the overlap between the covered stent and the cuff is usually 10-15 mm. Relining with an oversized bare stent may be required.
- The hydrophilic through-and-through wire guide is withdrawn before the stent is deployed.
- The introducer sheath of the graft is withdrawn until the external iliac component is fully deployed.
- To disconnect the proximal and distal attachment of the graft from the delivery system, remove sequentially the trigger-wires (Figure 7.10).
- The delivery system can then be removed. To avoid any dislodgement keep the balloon catheter in the bridging stent inflated.
- Kissing ballooning of both segments with a 10 mm or 12 mm balloon in the main body and with an 8 mm balloon in the side branch (Figure 7.11).

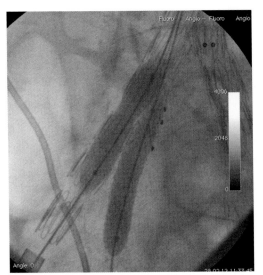

Figure 7.11 Two balloon catheters (12 mm for the main body and 8 mm for the hypogastric artery) are inflated in the side branch segments in a kissing balloon fashion to ensure patency of the EIA and IIA.

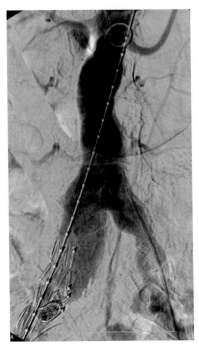

Figure 7.12 After the IBD has been implanted, the aortic aneurysm is repaired with a bifurcated Zenith AAA graft.

- If the abdominal aorta is involved (Figure 7.12), a bifurcated Zenith® AAA graft is introduced through the opposite iliac artery and deployed as usual (Figure 7.13).
- All the components have to be deployed with enough overlap to avoid late type III endoleak.
- A Zenith Iliac Leg graft (TFLE or ZSLE) with a distal diameter of 16 mm is implanted via the iliac bifurcation access site into the contralateral limb of the abdominal graft, connecting the lumen of the abdominal graft to the Branch Endovascular Graft-Iliac Bifurcation (Figure 7.14).
- Finally, a Zenith® Iliac Leg graft (TFLE or ZSLE) is deployed into the ipsilateral limb of the Zenith AAA graft.
- Completion angiography is performed to exclude endoleaks and to verify that the IIA is patent.
- Patency of the hypogastric artery and freedom from endoleak should be evaluated by yearly CT angiography (Figure 7.15). Figures 7.16-7.27 show the procedure step-by-step.

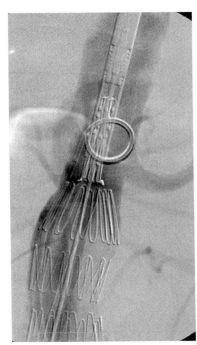

Figure 7.13 A bifurcated Zenith AAA graft is introduced through the opposite iliac artery and deployed as usual.

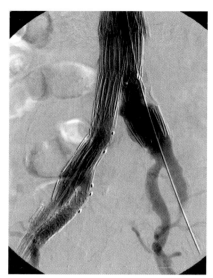

Figure 7.14 Through the IBD access site a Zenith Iliac Leg graft (16 mm distal diameter) is implanted into the contralateral limb of the abdominal graft, connecting the abdominal stent graft with the IBD. To avoid late type III endoleak, enough overlapping between the components is recommended. The second proximal marker helps identifying the origin of the hypogastric side branch. On the left side a Zenith Iliac Leg graft (ZSLE) is deployed into the ipsilateral limb of the Zenith AAA graft.

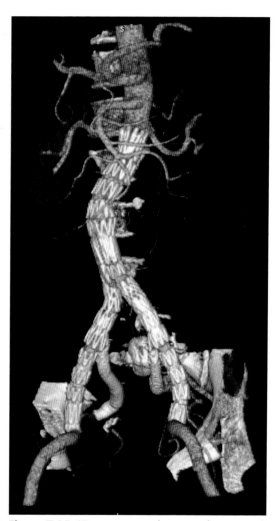

Figure 7.15 CT reconstruction after repair of an AAA with involvement of both common iliac arteries with iliac side branch endografts.

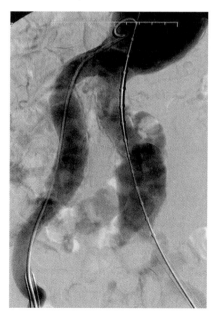

Figure 7.16 Angiography of a patient with an aneurysm of the infrarenal aorta and of both common iliac arteries.

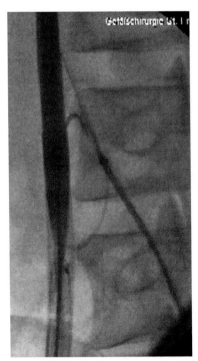

Figure 7.17 After fluoroscopic check of the position of the four radiopaque markers, the delivery system is advanced through the right side until the nose cone reaches the infrarenal aorta. By partially retracting the sheath the pre-curved indwelling catheter is now visible. It should be positioned just above the aortic bifurcation.

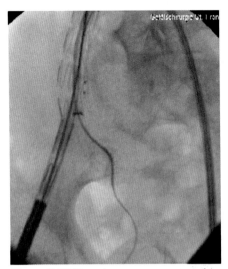

Figure 7.19 Through a separate puncture of the 12F sheath valve a catheter-guidewire combination is introduced into the IIA.

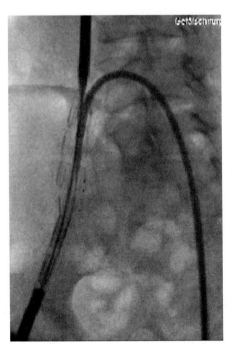

Figure 7.18 Through the indwelling catheter, a Terumo stiff guide wire is snared through a contralateral approach. A 12 F Flexor sheath is now advanced into the iliac side branch device.

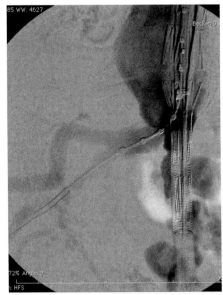

Figure 7.20 Selective angiography of the distal hypogastric artery. To visualize the distal landing zone, a different oblique projection is required for identification of the origin of the hypogastric artery. A graduated angiographic catheter is placed to estimate the length of the covered bridging stent.

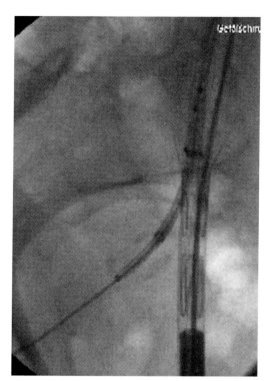

Figure 7.21 A 8x59 mm covered stent (Advanta V12, Atrium) preloaded in the 7F Flexor sheath is advanced into the hypogastric artery. Once the bridging stent is in place, the indwelling wire has to be removed.

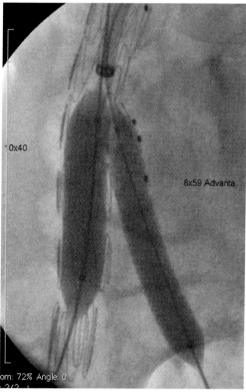

Figure 7.22 The Advanta covered stent is deployed with respect to the side branch overlap (14 mm) and the fixation site just above the origin of the first hypogastric branch. Kissing ballooning of the internal and external stented segment is now performed.

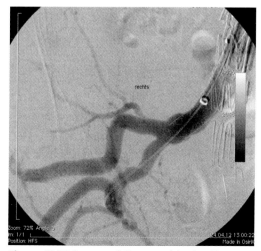

Figure 7.23 Because of dilatation of the distal hypogastric artery, wall apposition is not ideal.

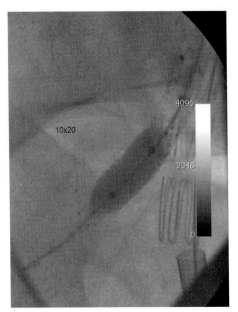

Figure 7.24 Relining of the covered stent with a large self-expanding bare metal stent (Zilver 10x40 mm) and ballooning with a 10x40 mm PTA catheter improve the distal wall apposition of the bridging stent.

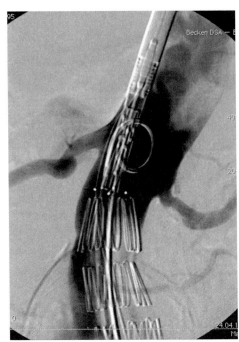

Figure 7.25 A bifurcated Zenith AAA graft is introduced through the left side and deployed as usual.

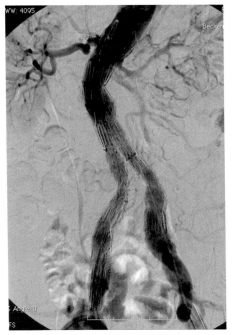

Figure 7.26 Completion angiography after implantation of the bifurcated Zenith AAA endograft showing a good patency of both renal arteries and no endoleak.

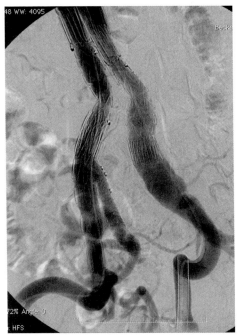

Figure 7.27 Angiography of the distal portion of the endograft showing exclusion of the aortoiliac aneurysm with good patency of both hypogastric arteries.

References

1. Pitoulias GA, Donas KP, Schulte S, *et al.* Isolated iliac artery aneurysms: endovascular versus open elective repair. J Vasc Surg 2007;46(4):648-54.
2. Malina M, Dirven M, Sonesson B, *et al.* Feasibility of a branched stent-graft in common iliac artery aneurysms. J Endovasc Ther 2006;13:496-500.
3. Serracino-Inglott F, Bray AE, Myers P. Endovascular abdominal aortic aneurysm repair in patients with common iliac artery aneurysms - Initial experience with the Zenith bifurcated iliac side branch device. J Vasc Surg 2007;46:211-7.
4. Haulon S, Greenberg RK, Pfaff K, *et al.* Branched grafting for aortoiliac aneurysms. Eur J Vasc Endovasc Surg. 2007;33:567-74.
5. Naik J, Hayes PD, Sadat U, *et al.* Internal iliac artery branch graft for common iliac artery aneurysm following previous open abdominal aortic aneurysm repair. Eur J Vasc Endovasc Surg 2008;35:436-8.
6. Coscas R, Greenberg RK, Pfaff K. Embolization of a type 2 endoleak through catheterization of a hypogastric branched stent-graft. J Vasc Surg 2010;51:712-4.
7. Ferreira M, Monteiro M, Lanziotti L. Technical aspects and midterm patency of iliac branch devices. J Vasc Surg 2010;51:545-50.
8. Pua U, Tan K, Rubin BB, *et al.* Iliac branch graft in the treatment of complex aortoiliac aneurysms: early results from a North American institution. J Vasc Inter Radiol 2011;22:542-49.
9. Donas KP, Torsello G, Pitoulias GA, *et al.* Surgical versus endovascular repair by iliac branch device of aneurysms involving the iliac bifurcation. J Vasc Surg 2011;53:1223-9.
10. Ziegler P, Avgerinos ED, Umscheid T, *et al.* Branched iliac bifurcation: 6 years experience with endovascular preservation of internal iliac artery flow. J Vasc Surg 2007;46:204-10.
11. Dias NV, Resch TA, Sonesson B, *et al.* EVAR of aortoiliac aneurysms with branched stent-grafts. Eur J Vasc Endovasc Surg 2008;35:677-84.
12. Tielliu IFJ, Bos WTGJ, Zeebregts CJ, *et al.* The role of branched endografts in preserving internal iliac arteries. J Cardiovasc Surg 2009;50:213-8.
13. Verzini F, Parlani G, Romano L, *et al.* Endovascular treatment of iliac aneurysm: concurrent comparison of side branch endograft versus hypogastric exclusion. J Vasc Surg 2009;49:1154-61.
14. Grenville J, Tan KT, Tse LW, *et al.* Bridging stent-graft pullout analysis. J Endovasc Ther 2011;18(2):161-8.

CHAPTER 8

Endovascular techniques for type B aortic dissection

G. Torsello, M. Austermann

The treatment of type B aortic dissection is challenging, and open surgery, particularly when performed under emergency conditions, continues to be associated with considerable mortality and morbidity rates.

Best medical treatment has been advocated as the first line therapy in patients without symptoms. In case of complications such as rupture (Figures 8.1, 8.2), end-organ ischemia (Figure 8.3), uncontrollable pain or hypertension, endovascular therapy is the treatment of choice in the overwhelming majority of patients.

Treatment strategy is individually based on anatomy and clinical manifestation.

In cases in which the implantation of a stent graft is indicated, exclusion of the primary entry tear is the main treatment goal, extending distally the stent-graft coverage if persistent false-lumen perfusion is demonstrated. The advantage of a more extensive coverage is to reduce long-term complications by excluding most reentry tears. On the other hand, with increasing aortic coverage, the risk of paraplegia also grows. Paraplegia after endografting is less common than after open surgery, but remains a significant concern after occlusion of the left subclavian artery and in patients with intraoperative and postoperative hypotension.

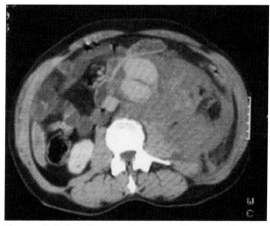

Figure 8.1 Type B aortic dissection with contained rupture of the thoracic aorta.

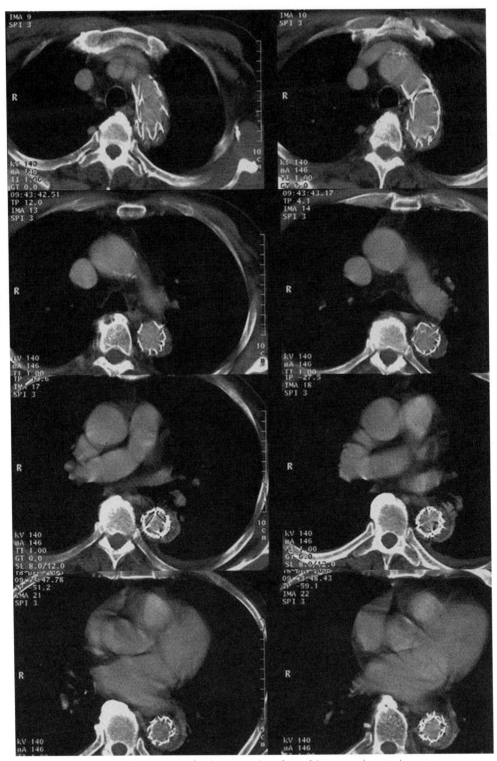

Figure 8.2 CT angiography one year after thoracic endografting of the ruptured aortic dissection.

Procedures

Aortic endografting

– Endograft implantation requires access through one common femoral artery. The need of a surgical conduit with a 10 mm graft is not frequent. However, it can facilitate access in patients with demanding iliac anatomy.

– Angiographic control can be achieved through a transbrachial or a contralateral femoral access. The first approach is preferred in patients with multiple reentries or complex anatomy for a better identification of the true lumen. Navigation of the stiff wire over an angiographic catheter should be done under fluoroscopy. Transesophageal ultrasound can be used for detecting correct positioning of the stiff wire in the true lumen (Figure 8.4). If necessary the "pig embracement technique" of two pigtail catheters, one through the brachial access and one from the femoral, can be used. Alternatively, segmental aortography through a long sheath can document the correct position of the wire already placed in the aortic arch.

– Over a stiff wire (Lunderqvist, Cook), the endograft is advanced into the aorta and placed at the level of the entry, usually at the origin of the left subclavian artery (Figure 8.5).

– To avoid aortic rupture and retrograde type A dissection, flexible grafts with a lower profile delivery system are preferred. As opposed to treatment strategies for thoracic aneurysms, minimal if any oversizing is necessary.

– For exact placement of the stent graft, lowering of the systolic blood pressure during the deployment is recommended. Endograft moulding with a balloon should be avoided.

– Left subclavian artery (LSA) coverage can increase the risk of stroke as well as para-

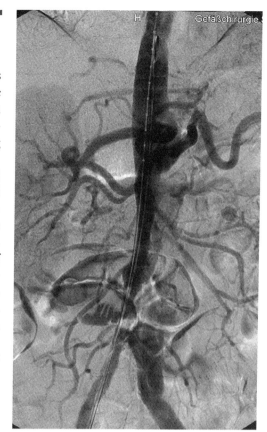

Figure 8.3 Type B aortic dissection with ischemia of the left kidney.

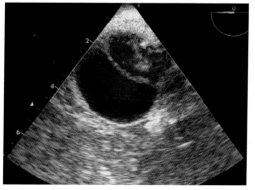

Figure 8.4 Transoesophageal imaging of the aortic dissection showing the true and false lumen as well as the wire in place.

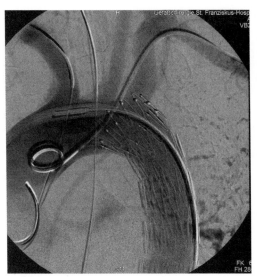

Figure 8.5 Treatment of the type B dissection with a TX2 Zenith stent graft with exclusion of the primary entry tear just below the origin of the left subclavian artery.

plegia, but can reduce the rate of proximal type I endoleak and false-lumen volume increase. Revascularization with subclavian-carotid transposition (Figures 8.6-8.8), carotid-to-subclavian bypass, or use of chimney and fenestrated grafts can reduce the risk of stroke, paraplegia and upper-limb ischemia if the left subclavian artery must be overstented.

– Completion angiography is performed to exclude endoleaks and document normal organ perfusion.

– In patients at high-risk for paraplegia (extended coverage of the aorta) CSF pressure has to be carefully monitored and corrected by CS fluid drainage (Figure 8.9).

Management of malperfusion syndromes

In some cases, stent-graft implantation can restore organ perfusion by remodelling the dissected aortic wall (Figures 8.10, 8.11).

If the malperfusion cannot be treated by aortic endografting alone, rapid restoration

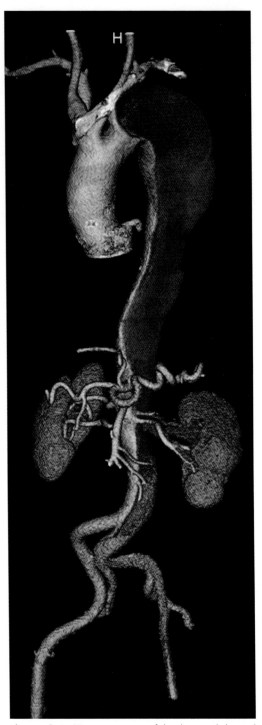

Figure 8.6 CT reconstruction of the thoracoabdominal aorta after type B aortic dissection. The entry is at level of the left subclavian artery, which was revascularized by transposition to the left common carotid artery.

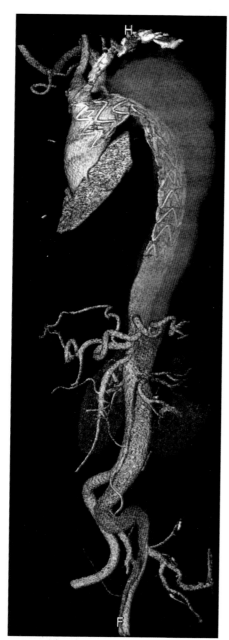

Figure 8.7 CT reconstruction after treatment with Valiant Captivia stent graft and subclavian-carotid transposition on the left side.

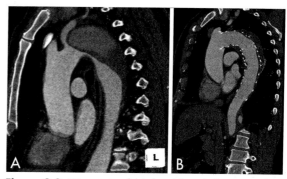

Figure 8.8 CT angiography before (A) and after stentgrafting (B) showing complete expansion of the true lumen and shrinkage of the false lumen.

of end-organ perfusion should be achieved by fen-estrations, balloon angioplasty, stenting of the occluded vessels or implantation of uncovered stents at or across the visceral aortic segment (petticoat concept). For this purpose we use a CE-marked nitinol dissection stent (Cook), along with the barbless TX2 as suggested by Lombardi et al. Timing and type of treatment for a given patient have to be customized on the basis of clinical status and CTA imaging.

Scissor technique

– Two rigid guide wires are introduced through the same femoral access, one into the true lumen and one into the false lumen. The study of

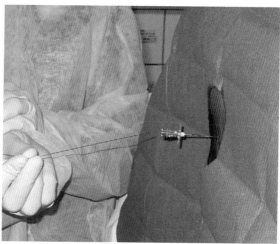

Figure 8.9 Lumbar puncture for placement of a spinal catheter for monitoring and correction of the CS fluid pressure.

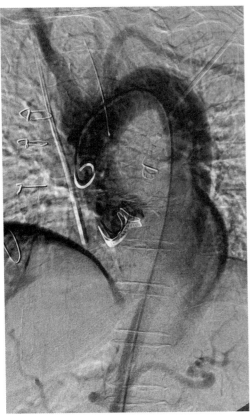

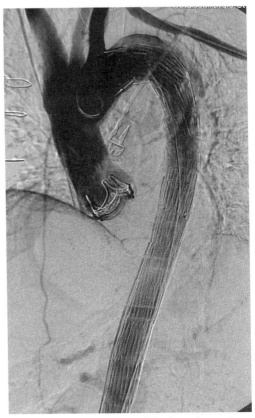

Figure 8.10 True lumen collapse with malperfusion involving the lower extremities and the right kidney.

Figure 8.11 Reconstitution of the flow after implantation of thoracic stent graft and bare metal stent (Zenith Dissection device) covering the aorta at the level of the visceral and renal vessels (petticoat concept).

the preoperative CTA and identification of the reentry can help for catheterization of the false lumen with an angled catheter-wire combination.

- Advancing one large, long sheath over the two wires should destroy the dissection lamella (Figure 8.12).
- After removing of the guide wire from the false lumen, a large balloon catheter is inflated in the true lumen and pulled back down to the aortic bifurcation. This manoeuvre is necessary because of the risk of creating an iatrogenic aortic coartation by pushing a rigid lamella which has not been completely cut.
- As an alternative procedure, a two groins approach can be used. One guide wire is passed from the true to the false lumen, snared with a goose neck catheter, and carefully pulled down to open the dissection membrane as wide as necessary (Figures 8.13-8.15).

Catheter-guided fenestration

The goal of the procedure is to create an artificial tear of the dissection flap at the origin of the occluded vessel, mitigating the dynamic obstruction (Figures 8.16-8.18). In case of rigidity of the lamella, the communication between the true and the false lumen is achieved using

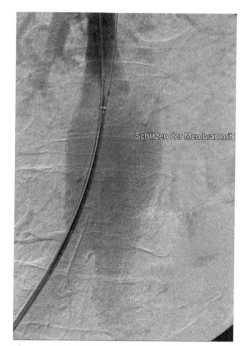

Figure 8.12 "Scissor technique". Over two stiff wires a long sheath is advanced into the aorta cutting the lamella.

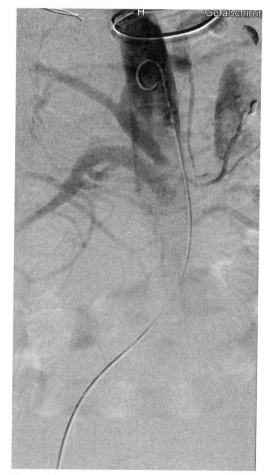

Figure 8.13 Angiography of patient with renal and lower extremities malperfusion caused by type B aortic dissection

a needle. A guide wire can then be advanced through the lamella into the lumen of the target vessel. In patients with chronic dissections, reentry systems as the Outback catheter (Cordis) or TIPS needle can be useful (Figures 8.19-8.24).

Adjunctive stenting (Figures 8.25, 8.26) may be necessary if PTA alone cannot sufficiently restore organ perfusion. Balloon-mounted stents are usually required for renal and visceral arteries, and self-expanding stents for the aorta and iliac arteries. Bare metal stents are preferred to preserve the perfusion of the lumbar and hypogastric arteries, lowering the risk of postoperative paraplegia.

Reperfusion syndrome after lower limb ischemia requires careful intensive monitoring and treatment for correcting postischemic metabolic misbalance. The potential need for fasciotomy or exploratory laparotomy must be taken into account.

A typical late complication of thoracoabdominal dissection is aneurysm formation at the level of an untreated false lumen. Fenestrated and branched endografts can be used for repair. However, the treatment is technically demanding (for details see Chapter 4, 5 and 6).

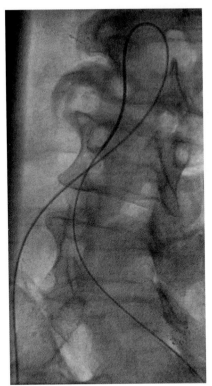

Figure 8.14 Alternatively to the scissor technique a guide wire has been passed from the true into the false lumen and snared with a goose neck catheter. Pulling on both ends of the guide wire the dissection membrane will be destroyed solving the malperfusion.

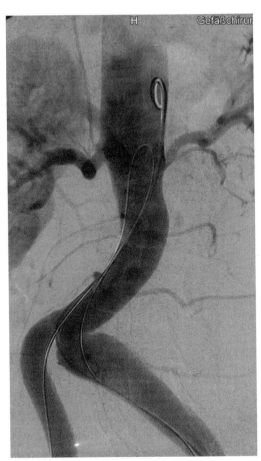

Figure 8.15 Angiography after bright fenestration of the dissection membrane.

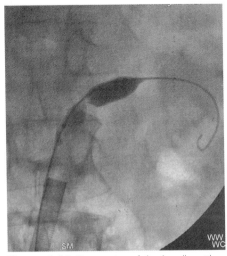

Figure 8.16 Fenestration of the lamella with a large balloon catheter. Note the narrowing at the level of the dissection membrane which disappears after the fenestration is completed.

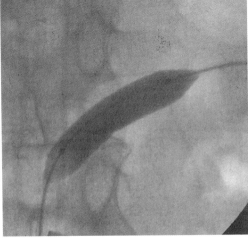

Figure 8.17 Fully expanded balloon catheter after the lamella has been destroyed.

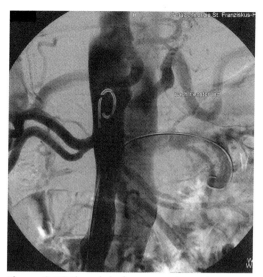

Figure 8.18 Through the fenestration the guide wire can be advanced into the left renal artery.

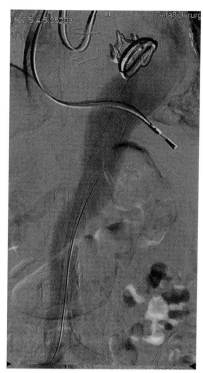

Figure 8.19 Angiography of a patient with chronic mesenteric ischemia four months after aortic dissection. No antegrade flow of the superior mesenteric artery could be detected.

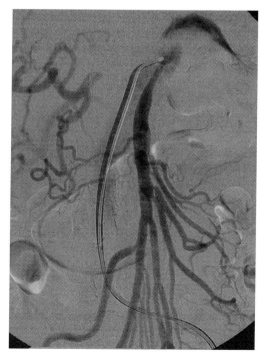

Figure 8.20 Through the false lumen selective angiography shows a normal morphology of the superior mesenteric artery.

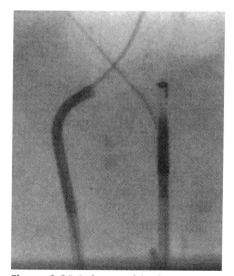

Figure 8.21 Perforation of the dissection membrane with the Out Back catheter (Cordis) with the same technique used for complete occlusion of the femoral or popliteal artery. The wire is snared with a goose neck catheter to advance a 6F sheath into the superior mesenteric artery.

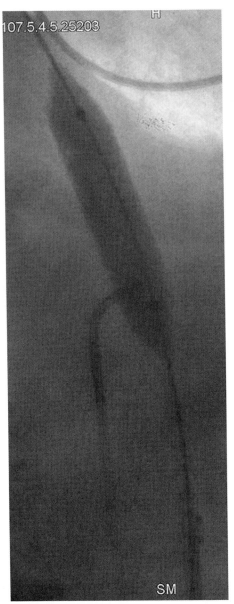

Figure 8.22 A large balloon catheter is in inflated to enlarge the fenestration.

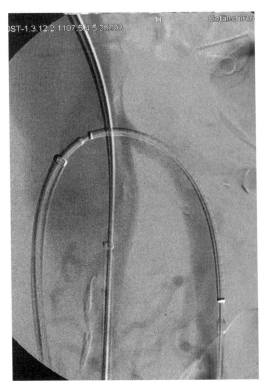

Figure 8.23 Through the sheath a self-expandable stent is used as bridging stent between the true lumen and the superior mesenteric artery.

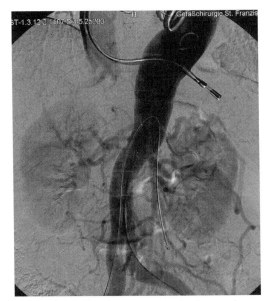

Figure 8.24 Completion angiography showing the antegrade flow of the superior mesenteric artery.

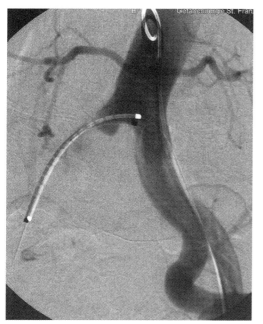

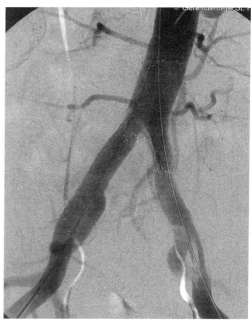

Figure 8.25 Complete occlusion of the right common iliac artery treated with stenting through cross-over approach.

Figure 8.26 Angiography after stenting of the right common iliac artery after flow restoration.

References

1. Dake MD, Miller DC, Mitchell RS. Endovascular stent-graft placement for the treatment of acute aortic dissection. N Engl J Med 1999:340:1524-31.
2. Nienaber CA, Kische S, Zeller T, *et al.* Provisional extension to induce complete attachment after stent-graft placement in type B aortic dissection: The PETTICOAT concept. J Endovasc Ther 2006;13:738-46.
3. Mossop PJ, McLachlan CS, Amukotuwa SA, *et al.* Staged endovascular treatment for complicated type B aortic dissection. Nat Clin Pract Cardiovasc Med 2005;2:316-22.
4. Peterson BG, Eskandari MK, Gleason TG, *et al.* Utility of left subclavian artery revascularization in association with endoluminal repair of acute and chronic thoracic aortic pathology. J Vasc Surg 2006;43:433-9.
5. Estrera AL, Miller CC 3rd, Safi HJ, *et al.* Outcomes of medical management of acute type B aortic dissection. Circulation 2006;114(Suppl 1):I384-9.
6. Viljanen T, Luosto R, Järvinen A, *et al.* Surgical treatment of aortic dissection. Scand Cardiovasc J 1986; 20:193-201.
7. Nienaber CA, Rousseau H, Eggebrecht H, *et al.* A randomized comparison of strategies for type B aortic dissection: The INvestigation of STEnt Grafts i Aortic Dissection (INSTEAD) Trial. Circulation 2009: 120:2519-28.
8. Eggebrecht H, *et al.* Endovascular stent-graft placement in aortic dissection: a meta-analysis. Circulation 2009;120:2519-28.
9. Resch TA, Delle M, Falkenberg M, *et al.* Remodeling of the thoracic aorta after stent grafting of type B dissection: A Swedish multicenter study. J Cardiovasc Surg 2006;47:503-8.
10. Manning BJ, Dias N, Manno M, *et al.* Endovascular treatment of acute complicated type B dissection. J Endovasc Ther 2009;16:466.
11. Yuan LX, Bao JM, Zhao ZQ, *et al.* Simultaneous multi-tear exclusion: An optimal strategy for type B thoracic aortic dissection initially proved by a single center's 8 years experience. Chin Med J 2007;120:2210-4.
12. Hinchliffe RJ, MacSweeney STR. Endovascular repair of a ruptured chronic type B aortic dissection J Vasc Surg 2002;36:401-3.

13. Cheung AT, Pochettino A, McGarvey ML, *et al.* Strategies to manage paraplegia risk after endovascular stent repair of descending thoracic aortic aneurysms. Ann Thorac Surg 2005;80:1280-8.

14. Atkins MD, Black JH, Cambria RP. Aortic dissection: perspectives in the era of stent-graft repair. J Vasc Surg 2006;43(Suppl A):30A-43.

15. Rodriguez JA, Olsen DM, Lucas L, *et al.* Aortic remodeling after endografting of thoracoabdominal aortic dissection. J Vasc Surg 2008;47:1188-94.

16. Kim U, Hong SJ, Kim J, *et al.* Intermediate to long-term outcomes of endoluminal stent-graft repair in patients with chronic type B aortic dissection. J Endovasc Ther 2009;16:42-7.

17. Feezor RJ, Martin TD, Hess PJ, *et al.* Early outcomes after endovascular management of acute, complicated type B aortic dissection. J Vasc Surg 2009;49:561-6.

18. Torsello GB, Torsello GF, Osada N, *et al.* The TRAVIATA registry of Valiant stent graft: Midterm results after treatment of diseases of the thoracic aorta. J Endovasc Ther 2010;17:137-50.

19. Lombardi JV, Cambria RP, Nienaber CA, *et al.* Prospective multicenter clinical trial (STABLE) on the endovascular treatment of complicated type B aortic dissection using a composite device design. J Vasc Surg 2012;55:629-40.

CHAPTER 9

Most frequent materials for endovascular aortic repair

F. Marquez de Azevedo, B. Berekoven

Given the complexity of the above described procedures, a wide variability of materials is necessary for successful aneurysm repair. A great range of wires, angiographic catheters, sheaths, stents and stent grafts should be in stock. Therefore, it is important to plan each procedure step by step and make sure that the needed materials are available. Sometimes, the surgeon has to face unexpected situations. Thus, it is also important to consider materials for bail-out in advance of a procedure. Complex aortic cases also require a dedicated environment and a well-trained team. Because of extensive fluoroscopy time the procedures should be performed in a hybrid operating room, where the operation (cut down, conduit implantation, conversion) can be done under the necessary sterile conditions. Endovascular procedures are frequently performed in close collaboration between vascular surgeon and interventionalists. Alternatively, vascular surgeons adequately trained in endovascular techniques, as in our department, will do the same job reducing the personal costs. Nurses are also faced with a lot of challenges in the new medical environment. These challenges include rapid advances in techniques, technologies and materials. Aortic endografting is surpassing conventional surgery and this evolution stresses our usual way to work in the operating room. Parallel to the endovascular specialist in the current medical environment, also the role of the endovascular assistant (EVA) will increase in the future. A standardized professional curriculum is underway. As a service to our readers, we provide lists of the most frequent materials used for the described techniques. These lists do not include basic materials, which should be in storage in every hospital that performs endovascular procedures (Tables 9.I-9.V).

Company references

AngioDynamics, Queensbury, NY, USA
Atrium Medical corporation, Hudson, NH, USA
Cook Medical Inc., Bloomington, IN, USA
C.R. Bard Inc., Murray Hill, NJ, USA

ev3, Plymouth, MN, USA
Medtronic Vascular, Santa Rosa, CA, USA
Terumo Medical Corporation, Tokyo, Japan
W.L. Gore & Assoc. Inc., Flagstaff, AZ, USA

Table 9.1 Special endovascular equipment for chimney technique*

	Product	Company	Order number
1.	Radiofocus Introducer 5 F .035" 10 cm	Terumo	RS*B50K10MQ
2.	Radiofocus Introducer 8 F .035" 10 cm	Cook	RS*B80K10MQ
3.	Flexor Shuttle Sheath Introducer 6 F 90 cm .038" Straight	Cook	KSAW-6.0-38-90-RB-SHTL-Flex-HC
4.	Flexor Shuttle Sheath Introducer 7 F. 90 cm .038" Straight	Cook	KSAW-7.0-38-90-RB-SHTL-HC
5.	Flexor Sheath 7 F 110 cm .035" ANL1 Configuration	Cook	KCFW-7.0-35-110-RB-HFANL1-HC
6.	Flexor Sheath 8 F 110 cm .035" ANL1 Configuration	Terumo	KCFW-8.0-35-110-RB-HFANL1-HC
7.	Check Flow Sheath 14 F 13 cm .038"	Cook	RCF-14.0-38-J
8.	Lunderqvist Extra Stiff Guide Wire .035" 260 cm	Cook	TSCMG-35-260-7-LES
9.	Radiofocus Guide Wire M 035", 260 cm Standard	Terumo	RF*GA35263M
10.	Radiofocus Guide Wire M 035", 260 cm Stiff	Terumo	RF-PA35263M
11.	Starter Guide Wire.035" 180 cm J-Tip	Boston	49-120
12.	Rosen Guide Wire 260 cm .035", 260 cm J-Tip	Cook	THSCF-35-260-1.5-Rosen
13.	Calibration Catheter 5 F .035" 100 cm	Cook	NR5.0-35-100-P-10S-PIG-CSC-20
14.	Angiography Catheter Pigtail 5 F .035" 110 cm	Cordis	451-503L5
15.	Angiography Catheter Multipurpose A2(I) 5.2 F .038" 125 cm	Cordis	533-587
16.	Angiography Catheter Vertebral 5 F .038" 100 cm	Terumo	RF-YH15110M
17.	Angiography Catheter Shuttle Select SlipHink-Headhunter 6.5 F .035" 125 cm	Cook	SCBR6.5-35-125-P-NS-H1-SHTL
18.	Angiographie Catheter Headhunter H1 5 F .035" 100 cm	Boston	31-415
19.	Support Catheter Quick-Cross 5F .035" 135 cm, 45° Tip angled	Spectranetics	518-081
20.	Reliant Stent Graft Balloon Catheter 46 mm 8 F 100 cm	Medtronic	AB46
21.	Prostar XL 10 F monorail percutan Close System	Abbott	12322
22.	Vascular V12 Advanta Covered Stentgraft .035" 120 cm working length	Atrium	various sizes (6×22,6×38,6×59,7×22,7× 38,7×58,8×22,8×38,8×59) mm
23.	Viabahn Endoprothesis with Propaten Surface .035" 120 cm working length	Gore	various sizes (7×10,8×5,8×10,8×15,10×5,1 0×10,10×15,13×5,13×10) mm/cm
24.	Smart Control self-expandable Nitinol Stent .035" 120 cm working length	Cordis	various sizes (7×40,7×60,7×80,8×40,8× 60,8×80,10×40,10×60,10×80) mm
25.	Zilver Flex self-expandable Nitinol Stent .035" 125 cm working length	Cook	various sizes (8×40,8×60,8×80,10× 40,10×60,10×80) mm

* Information without guarantee.

Table 9.II Special endovascular equipment for ISB technique*

	Product	Company	Order number
1.	Radiofocus Introducer 5 F .035" 10 cm	Terumo	RS*B50K10MQ
2.	Radiofocus Introducer 8 F .035" 10 cm	Terumo	RS*B80K10MQ
3.	Flexor Shuttle Sheath Introducer 7 F 90 cm .038" Straight	Cook	KSAW-7.0-38-90-RB-SHTL-HC
4.	Flexor Sheath 7 F 110 cm .035" ANL1 Configuration	Cook	KCFW-7.0-35-110-RB-HFANL1-HC
5.	Flexor Sheath 12 F 45 cm .035" ANL1 Configuration	Cook	RCFW-12.0-35-45-RB-HFANL1-HC
6.	Check Flow Sheath 14 F 13 cm .038"	Cook	RCF-14.0-38-J
7.	Lunderqvist Extra Stiff Guide Wire .035" 260 cm	Cook	TSCMG-35-260-7-LES
8.	Radiofocus Guide Wire M 035", 260 cm Standard	Terumo	RF*GA35263M
9.	Radiofocus Guide Wire M 035", 260 cm Stiff	Terumo	RF-PA35263M
10.	Starter Guide Wire .035" 180 cm J-Tip	Boston	49-120
11.	Rosen Guide Wire 260 cm .035", 260 cm J-Tip	Cook	THSCF-35-260-1.5-Rosen
12.	Calibration Catheter 5 F .035" 100 cm	Cook	NR5.0-35-100-P-10S-PIG-CSC-20
13.	Angiographie Catheter Pigtail 5 F .035" 90 cm	Cordis	451-503F5
14.	Angiography Catheter Multipurpose A2(I) 5.2 F .038" 125 cm	Cordis	533-587
15.	Angiographie Catheter Vertebral 5F .038" 100 cm	Terumo	RF-YH15110M
16.	Indy otw Vascular Retriever System	Cook	INDY-8.0-35-100-40
17.	Prostar XL 10F monorail percutan Close System	Abbott	12322
18.	Vascular V12 Advanta Covered Stentgraft .035" 120 cm working length	Atrium	various sizes (7x38,7x59,8x22,8x38,8x59) mm
19.	Viabahn Endoprothesis with Propaten Surface .035" 120 cm working length	Gore	various sizes (7x10,8x5,8x10,8x15) mm/cm
20.	Smart Control self-expandable Nitinol Stent .035" 120 cm working length	Cordis	various sizes (7×40,7×60,7×80,8× 40,8×60,8×80) mm
21.	Zilver Flex self-expandable Nitinol Stent .035" 125 cm working length	Cook	various sizes (8×40,8×60,8×80) mm

* Information without guarantee.

Table 9.III Special endovascular equipment for branched technique*

	Product	Company	Order number
1.	Radiofocus Introducer 5 F .035" 10 cm	Terumo	RS*B50K10MQ
2.	Radiofocus Introducer 8 F .035" 10 cm	Terumo	RS*B80K10MQ
3.	Flexor Shuttle Sheath Introducer 6 F. 90 cm .038" Straight	Cook	KSAW-6.0-38-90-RB-SHTL-Flex-HC
4.	Flexor Shuttle Sheath Introducer 7 F. 90 cm .038" Straight	Cook	KSAW-7.0-38-90-RB-SHTL-HC
5.	Flexor Sheath 7 F 110 cm .035" ANL1 Configuration	Cook	KCFW-7.0-35-110-RB-HFANL1-HC
6.	Flexor Sheath 12 F 45 cm .035" ANL1 Configuration	Cook	RCFW-12.0-35-45-RB-HFANL1-HC
7.	Check Flow Sheath 14 F 13 cm .038"	Cook	RCF-14.0-38-J
8.	Extra Large Check-Flow Introducer 22 F .038" 30 cm	Cook	XLCFW-22.0-38-30-ENDOSTENT
9.	Lunderqvist Extra Stiff Guide Wire .035" 260 cm	Cook	TSCMG-35-260-7-LES
10.	Radiofocus Guide Wire M 035", 260 cm Standard	Terumo	RF*GA35263M
11.	Radiofocus Guide Wire M 035", 260 cm Stiff	Terumo	RF-PA35263M
12.	Starter Guide Wire.035" 180 cm J-Tip	Boston	49-120
13.	Rosen Guide Wire 260 cm .035", 260 cm J-Tip	Cook	THSCF-35-260-1.5-Rosen
14.	Calibration Catheter 5 F .035" 100 cm	Cook	NR5.0-35-100-P-10S-PIG-CSC-20
15.	Angiography Catheter Pigtail 5 F .035" 90 cm	Cordis	451-503F5
16.	Angiography Catheter SHK 0.8 5 F .035" 65 cm	Boston	31-481
17.	Angiography Catheter Vertebral 5 F .038" 100 cm	Terumo	RF-YH15110M
18.	Angiography Catheter Cobra (2) 5 F .038" 100 cm	Terumo	RF-XB55110M
19.	Angiography Catheter Headhunter H1 5 F .035" 100 cm	Boston	31-415
20.	Angiography Catheter Bernstein 5F .038" 100 cm	Cordis	451-513H0
21.	Angiography Catheter SOS Omni selectiv(3) 5 F .035" 80 cm	Angio Dynamics	10720404
22.	Support Catheter Quick-Cross 5 F .035" 135 cm, 45° Tip angled	Spectranetics	518-081
23.	Prostar XL 10F monorail percutan Close System	Abbott	12322
21.	Vascular V12 Advanta Covered Stentgraft .035" 120 cm working length	Atrium	various sizes (7x22,7x38,7x59,8x22,8x 38,8x59) mm
22.	Fluency Plus Vascular Stent Graft 117 cm working length	Bard	various sizes (8x40,8x60,8x80,10x40, 10x60,10x80) mm
23.	Smart Control self-expandable Nitinol Stent .035" 120 cm working length	Cordis	various sizes (7x40,7x60,7x80,8x40,8x 60,8x80,10x40,10x60,10x80) mm
24.	Zilver Flex self-expandable Nitinol Stent .035" 125 cm working length	Cook	various sizes (8x40,8x60,8x80,10x 40.10x60,10x80) mm
25.	Fluency Stentgraft	Bard	
26.	Smart Control Stent	Cordis	

* Information without guarantee.

Table 9.IV Special endovascular equipment for fenestrated technique*

	Product	Company	Order number
1.	Radiofocus Introducer 5 F .035" 10 cm	Terumo	RS*B50K10MQ
2.	Radiofocus Introducer 8 F .035" 10 cm	Terumo	RS*B80K10MQ
3.	Flexor Sheath 6 F .18"/.038" 55 cm ANL1 Configuration	Cook	KSAW-6.0-18/38-55-RB-ANL1-HC
4.	Flexor Sheath 6 F .18"/.038" 55 cm ANL2 Configuration	Cook	KSAW-6.0-18/38-55-RB-ANL2-HC
5.	Flexor Sheath 7 F .18"/.038" 55 cm ANL1 Configuration	Cook	KSAW-7.0-18/38-55-RB-ANL1-HC
6.	Flexor Sheath 7 F .18"/.038" 55 cm ANL2 Configuration	Cook	KSAW-7.0-18/38-55-RB-ANL2-HC
7.	Check Flow Sheath 14 F .038" 13 cm	Cook	RCF-14.0-38-J
8.	Extra Large Check-Flow Introducer 22 F .038" 30 cm	Cook	XLCFW-22.0-38-30-ENDOSTENT
9.	Lunderqvist Extra Stiff Guide Wire .035" 260 cm	Cook	TSCMG-35-260-7-LES
10.	Radiofocus Guide Wire M 035", 260 cm Standard	Terumo	RF*GA35263M
11.	Radiofocus Guide Wire M 035", 260 cm Stiff	Terumo	RF-PA35263M
12.	Starter Guide Wire .035" 180 cm J-Tip	Boston	49-120
13.	Rosen Guide Wire 260 cm .035",260 cm J-Tip	Cook	THSCF-35-260-1.5-Rosen
14.	Calibration Catheter 5 F .035" 100 cm	Cook	NR5.0-35-100-P-10S-PIG-CSC-20
15.	Angiography Catheter Pigtail 5 F .035" 90 cm	Cordis	451-503F5
16.	Angiography Catheter SHK 0.8 5 F .035" 65 cm	Boston	31-481
17.	Angiography Catheter Vertebral 5 F .038" 100 cm	Terumo	RF-YH15110M
18.	Angiography Catheter Cobra (2) 5 F .038" 100 cm	Terumo	RF-XB55110M
19.	Angiography Catheter Bernstein 5 F .038" 100 cm	Cordis	451-513H0
20.	Angiographie Catheter SOS Omni selectiv(3) 5 F .035" 80 cm	Angio Dynamics	10720404
21.	Support Catheter Quick-Cross 5F .035" 135cm, 45° Tip angled	Spectranetics	518-081
22.	Prostar XL 10 F monorail percutan Close System	Abbott	12322
23.	Vascular V12 Advanta Covered Stentgraft .035" 120 cm working length	Atrium	various sizes (6×22,6×38,7×22,7× 38,8×22,8×38) mm
24.	Palmaz Genesis Balloon expandable Stent .035" 135 cm working length	Cordis	various sizes (6×18,6×24,6×29,7× 18,7×24,7×29) mm
25.	V 12 Advanta Stentgraft.035"	Atrium	
26.	Palmaz Genesis .035"	Cordis	

* Information without guarantee.

Table 9.V Special endovascular equipment for Typ B-Aortic Dissection*

	Product	Company	Order number
1.	Radiofocus Introducer 5 F .035" 10 cm	Terumo	RS*B50K10MQ
2.	Radiofocus Introducer 8 F .035" 10 cm	Terumo	RS*B80K10MQ
3.	Flexor Shuttle Sheath Introducer 6 F. 90 cm .038" Straight	Cook	KSAW-6.0-38-90-RB-SHTL-Flex-HC
4.	Flexor Shuttle Sheath Introducer 7 F. 90 cm .038" Straight	Cook	KSAW-7.0-38-90-RB-SHTL-HC
5.	Check Flow Sheath 14 F. 13 cm .038"	Cook	RCF-14.0-38-J
6.	Lunderqvist Extra Stiff Guide Wire .035" 260 cm double curved	Cook	TSCMG-35-260-7-LESDC
7.	Radiofocus Guide Wire M 035", 260 cm Standard	Terumo	RF*GA35263M
8.	Radiofocus Guide Wire M 035", 260 cm Stiff	Terumo	RF-PA35263M
9.	Starter Guide Wire .035" 180 cm J-Tip	Boston	49-120
10.	Calibration Catheter 5 F .035" 100 cm	Cook	NR5.0-35-100-P-10S-PIG-CSC-20
11.	Angiography Catheter Pigtail 5 F .035" 110 cm	Cordis	451-503L5
12.	Angiography Catheter SHK 0.8 5 F .035" 65 cm	Boston	31-481
13.	Angiography Catheter Vertebral 5 F .038" 100 cm	Terumo	RF-YH15110M
14.	Angiography Catheter Cobra (2) 5 F .038" 100 cm	Terumo	RF-XB55110M
15.	Angiography Catheter SOS Omni selectiv (3) 5 F .035" 80 cm	Angio Dynamics	10720404
16.	Outback LTD Re-Entry System 6 F 120 cm working length	Cordis	OTB42121
17.	Reliant Stent Graft Balloon Catheter 46 mm 8F 100 cm	Medtronic	AB46
18.	Prostar XL 10F monorail percutan Close System	Abbott	12322
19.	Zenith TX2 Thoracic Endograft Low Profile	Cook	various sizes (xx) mm
20.	Zenith Dissection Endovascular Stent	Cook	various sizes (46x82,46x123,46x164) mm
21.	E-XL Aortic self-expandable Stent	Jotec	various sizes (20x100,24x100,28x 130,32x130,36x130) mm
22.	Vascular V12 Advanta Covered Stentgraft .035" 120 cm working length	Atrium	various sizes (7x22,7x38,7x59,8x22,8x38,8x59) mm
23.	Palmaz Genesis Balloon expandable Stent .035" 135 cm working length	Cordis	various sizes (6x18,6x24,6x29,7x18,7 x24,7x29) mm
24.	Smart Control self-expandable Nitinol Stent .035" 120 cm working length	Cordis	various sizes (7x40,7x60,7x80,8x40,8x 60,8x80,) mm
25.	V 12 Advanta Stentgraft.035"	Atrium	

* Information without guarantee.

CHAPTER 10

Evolution of vascular and endovascular surgery in the 21ᵗʰ century from the point of view of a young vascular surgeon

K.P. Donas

"…death of a species is a consequence
of non-adaptation to changing circumstances…"
Charles Darwin

Almost 15 years ago (1997), the presidential address from Professor Frank J. Veith in the Journal of Vascular Surgery related Darwin´s theory to the evolution of Vascular Surgery. There is no doubt that in the past 20 years there is an ongoing change in the medical environment. The introduction of less-invasive catheter-guidewire-imaging techniques in the treatment of vascular diseases release fireworks of a possible safe alternative to the standard surgical approach.

The initial skepticism of the "traditional" vascular surgeons about this alternative approach was replaced with an increasing enthusiasm based on the profound belief that these less-invasive techniques will expand their role in the treatment of vascular disorders and eventually will replace the standardized surgical modalities. During this process there was a strength competition of Vascular Surgery with other nonsurgical interventional specialties such as Interventional Radiology and Cardiology. Additionally, Vascular Surgery came to be a separate specialty when it became obvious that general and cardiothoracic surgeons were not achieving optimal results with vascular operations. The need of a profound view of the vascular disease not only in the treatment but also in the prevention with synchronous inclusion of endovascular modalities in the therapeutic armamentarium led to a paradigm shift towards exclusive vascular operators.

Veith's suggestion that Vascular Surgery recognize that its specialty is not immutable or fixed by some Creative Power, but must constantly evolve to survive has been proven; Vascular Surgery has demonstrated remarkable adaptability in the modern era of endovascular treatment. Thus, as Darwin showed, transmutation of species is the rule and several current species or specialties may descend from a common ancestor (in our case General Surgery) to become clearly defined and separate specialties. In the last two decades, vascular surgeons have shown the ability to adapt and acquire endovascular skills giving them a protagonist role in the plethora of specialties with vascular interest.

Especially, over the last 20 years vascular surgeons showed a sustained improvement of the competence and professionalism with the catheter-guidewire-imaging techniques. In the meanwhile, endovascular options have been proven as safe and feasible in several clinical entities. However, aneurysms with hostile anatomies for procedure-related complications such as endoleaks, limb occlusions, lost of target vessels remain a challenge in the endovascular field. For this reason, there is an increasing need to present a modern guide with all important advanced endovascular approaches in order to standardize the techniques and give a significant impetus for further improvement and modification.

Personally, it is a great honour for me to be co-author of the present guide and I would like to express my deep thanks to Professor Dr. Giovanni Torsello for this. Finally, I would like to dedicate the present work to my father Dr. Perikles Donas, vascular surgeon, who is still the biggest inspiration for me.

PRINTED BY EDIZIONI MINERVA MEDICA - SEPTEMBER 2012 - SALUZZO (ITALY) - CORSO IV NOVEMBRE, 29-31